£12.99

The nutrition of older adults

The nutrition of older adults

Geoffrey P. Webb BSc, MSc, PhD

Senior Lecturer in Nutrition and Physiology, University of East London, UK

June Copeman BSc, MSc, MEd, SRD

Senior Lecturer in Nutrition and Dietetics, Leeds Metropolitan University, UK

A member of the Hodder Headline Group

LONDON • SYDNEY • AUCKLAND

First published in Great Britain in 1996 by
Arnold, a member of Hodder Headline Group,
338 Euston Road, London NW1 3BH

Co-published with Age Concern England, Astral House
1268 London Road, London SW16 4EJ

British Library Cataloguing in Publication Data
A catalogue record for this book is available from the British Library

ISBN 0 340 60156 6

Typeset in 10/12 pt Palatino by GreenGate Publishing Services, Tonbridge, Kent
Printed and bound in Great Britain by J.W. Arrowsmith Ltd., Bristol

Contents

Preface

About one in five of all UK adults is over the age of 65 years. There is also a considerable body of evidence which indicates that overt nutritional problems are far more prevalent amongst this age group than in any other section of the adult population. Despite this, most nutrition texts devote only a few pages to dealing with the particular nutritional needs, priorities and problems of older people. There are several texts about 'nutrition and the elderly' but these tend to be multi-author compilations of highly specialised papers or review articles that are often rather impenetrable for the non specialist reader.

This book is written with the non-specialist in mind and focuses specifically upon the nutritional needs and priorities of older people and upon those factors that may affect the food choices and nutritional status of older people. The book is intended to be a general, wide-ranging and readable introduction to the nutrition of elderly people for students and practitioners from a variety of academic and professional backgrounds, including: doctors, nurses and other health workers, nutritionists and dietitians, community care workers, health promotion officers, and managers with responsibility for the provision of services for the elderly. Given this varied readership, we have tried to write in a way that does not assume too much background knowledge of nutrition or the related scientific disciplines.

We would hope that this book would make some contribution to increasing awareness of the importance of good nutrition to the wellbeing of older people and raise the priority given to research and education in this field.

We would like to thank Dr Diane Jakobson for first suggesting the idea of writing a book on this topic. Her very thorough market research clearly identified the need for a book of this type and was critical in getting this project underway. We would also like to thank Mr Richard Holloway, formerly of Arnold now of Age Concern, for his advice, support and encouragement during the preparation of the manuscript.

Defining and describing the elderly population

Aims and scope of the chapter

In this chapter there is a brief overview of the effects of ageing and some of the implications of these age-related changes. We have tried to describe the elderly population in terms of:

- current and projected size
- mortality and morbidity
- gender and ethnic mix
- economic and social characteristics.

The elderly are a large and growing section of the population, they absorb a disproportionately large amount of health and social spending, and yet they are a disadvantaged section of the population in terms of health, economic status and 'social health'.

This discussion should add weight to the argument that the nutrition of the elderly, and indeed all aspects of health care and promotion in the elderly, deserves a higher priority. It makes economic sense, as well as being desirable upon humanitarian grounds, to research and develop nutrition education and health promotion strategies for the elderly. Any dietary improvements or other health promotion measures that maintain the health of the elderly population should lessen their dependence and reduce the costs of care. Such measures could also increase their capacity to contribute to the economy of the country, for example by continuing to work full or part-time, by doing socially desirable work on a voluntary basis, by following an economically productive hobby or interest, by minding children to allow younger relatives to work, or by simply being a readily available reservoir of knowledge and experience. A large population of relatively fit, experienced and well-educated over 65-year-olds, freed from the requirements of a conventional job but still seeking to use their extended retirement productively, could be an economic and social asset to a nation. This could offset some of the costs that inevitably result from the increasing numbers of dependent elderly.

Sections of this chapter might appear superficially to have limited relevance to a book about nutrition: for instance those sections dealing with the economic and social circumstances of the elderly and those looking at the differences in health problems of young and old. However, there is an abundance of evidence that social, economic and medical factors are major influences upon the food selection practices and nutritional status of older people.

Effects of ageing: an overview

Ageing is characterised by a gradual decline in the ability of an organism to adapt to environmental stresses and an inability to maintain homeostasis. Thus, for example, ageing of the immune system leads to a decline in the efficiency of the immune surveillance and defensive mechanisms which leads to increased incidence of infection, autoimmune disease and cancer (Kay, 1985). More generally, this loss of adaptability or capacity to maintain homeostasis results in increasing mortality rates, increased morbidity and increased rates of disability.

Figure 1.1 gives a quantitative illustration of how the mortality rate amongst British adults rises exponentially with age; less than 0.1% of men in the 25–34 age group die each year; this rises to about 4% in the 65–74s and to almost 20% in men over 85 years. Figure 1.2 shows how the self-reported health status of UK adults worsens with age. The number of people who perceive their health as good or very good declines with age and those perceiving their health as only fair or bad increases. Expectation presumably has an effect upon this perception and thus this figure might well underestimate the real decline in wellbeing with age because of declining expectations. Figure 1.3 shows estimates of the prevalence of disability amongst British adults of different ages. Once again, there is an exponential rise in rates of disability (of all severities) with age.

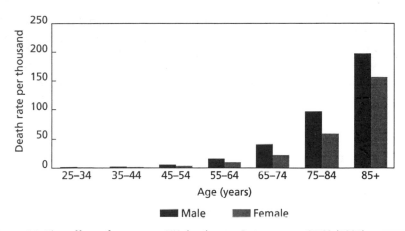

Figure 1.1 The effect of age upon UK death rate. Data source: OPCS (1991)

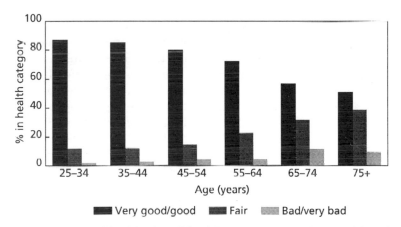

Figure 1.2 Self-reported health of English adults. Data source: White *et al.* (1993)

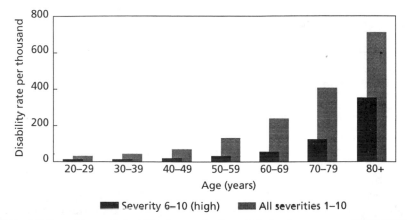

Figure 1.3 Prevalence of disability by age in Great Britain. Data source: OPCS (1988)

Figures 1.1 to 1.3 clearly demonstrate the deleterious effects of ageing upon morbidity and mortality rates. However, the rate of ageing is variable: in Figure 1.2, for example, around half of the over 75s still described their health as good or very good and only about 10% considered it to be bad or very bad. The rate of ageing is determined by both genetic and environmental factors; diet/nutritional status is one of numerous environmental factors that would be expected to influence the rate at which an individual ages.

A shortage of information on nutrition in the elderly

In recent years, there has been much attention given to developing nutrition education and related health promotion guidelines for the whole adult population. If implemented by younger adults, these guidelines would be expected to delay the age-related increases in mortality and morbidity outlined above. There has, however, been much less consideration of how the nutritional needs and priorities of older people might differ from those of younger adults. This book will focus upon those differences and hopefully indicate how general nutrition education guidelines might benefit from modification or re-interpretation when applied specifically to the older adult.

Monitoring the health and nutrition of elderly people generally seems to have been given relatively low priority in the UK in the recent past; frustratingly, 65 years is the age at which many health and/or nutrition surveys of the adult population seem to stop. For example, *The dietary and nutritional survey of British adults* (Gregory et al., 1990), the most recent nutritional survey of British adults, excluded persons over 65 years. The last major nutritional survey of the elderly population in the UK was conducted nearly 30 years ago in 1967/8 (DHSS, 1972) with a follow up survey of about half of the original sample in 1972/3 (DHSS, 1979). In the preface to the report on *The nutrition of elderly adults* (COMA, 1992) the chairman of COMA reports that 'all too often the work of the Group was constrained by lack of data'. This group made more than 20 recommendations for further investigation and research. We have also been constrained by this lack of data: our discussion of each of the key questions listed below has been severely hampered by lack of reliable data obtained directly from studies with elderly people.

- How do requirements for some nutrients change as people become elderly?
- Do biochemical and other standards of nutritional adequacy derived from studies with younger adults always remain appropriate in the old and very old?
- Does survey data obtained from younger adults reliably reflect the contribution of different foods to the supply of key nutrients in the elderly?
- How do nutrient intakes of elderly people compare with those of younger adults and thus how prevalent are nutritional inadequacies amongst the elderly population?
- Do disease 'risk factors' like overweight and serum cholesterol have the same predictive value in the elderly and thus are the guidelines aimed at reducing them equally valid in the elderly?

During the lifetime of this edition there will hopefully be significant improvement in this situation. In the *Health survey for England 1991* (White *et al.*, 1993), the sample population does include free-living people over 65 years. Although these authors note the lack of data on the over 65s from previous reports for comparison, the intention is that these health surveys will now be published annually and thus build up into a major database. At the time of writing, a major dietary survey of the elderly in Britain is in progress and it is due to be published in 1997 (Hughes *et al.*, 1995); this should provide good, up-to-date information on the dietary habits, nutritional status and nutrient intakes of elderly Britons.

When do adults become elderly?

Ageing is a continuous process that occurs throughout adult life and so before one can discuss the health and nutrition of elderly adults one must first decide what one means by elderly. The risks of both mortality and disability increase in a roughly exponential way throughout adult life due to the progressive loss of adaptability (Figures 1.1 to 1.3). Nevertheless, any cut-off points used to define the elderly are bound to be arbitrary because ageing occurs at different rates in different individuals and even in different physiological systems within the same individual (Evans, 1991). It is both illogical and unscientific to suggest that on their 65th, 75th or even 85th birthday, all people suddenly enter a different category. Although, on average, 70-year-olds are less 'fit' than 50 year olds and have a lower life expectancy, some people of 70 years will be physiologically younger than some people of 50 years and some 70-year-olds can expect to live longer than some 50-year-olds.

At the time of writing (early 1994) there has been considerable adverse comment in the UK press about the apparent rationing of specialist medical and surgical treatments on the arbitrary basis of chronological age. Evans (1991) argues forcefully for the integration of geriatric medicine with other medical specialisms and for the allocation of resources on the basis of physiology rather than age; some expensive treatments used in younger people are less cost effective than those that may be denied to older patients.

Despite accepting this individuality in the rates of ageing, we nonetheless feel the need to make some arbitrary division of people into age groups. Much of nutrition surveillance and education deals with population norms and population level interventions. Most of the current nutrition education guidelines in industrialised countries are based upon epidemiology – 'the study of the distribution and determinants of disease in human populations'. When dealing with *populations* then, the use of arbitrary age divisions is more acceptable and rational than using them to decide upon the most appropriate treatment for an *individual*.

The World Health Organization uses the following classification of age groups: 45–59, middle age; 60–74, elderly; 75–89, old; and, 90+, very old. We have taken 65 years as the nominal starting point for elderly people because this is so widely viewed as the defining point for the start of old age. It is the

Table 1.1 The percentage of the population of England and Wales in various age bands. Data source: OPCS (1993)

Age band	% of total population*
0–14 (children)	19.2
15–44 (young adults)	43.0
45–64 (middle-aged)	21.9
65+ (elderly adults)	15.9
65–74	8.8
75–84	5.4
85–89	1.2
90+	0.5

*total population of 51.3 million in 1992.

normal age of retirement for males in the UK. Where we have used subdivisions of the elderly population we have tended to take the 10 year bands 65–74 years and 75–84 years, with the over 85s regarded as a single category at the extreme of the range.

Table 1.1 shows the current age distribution of the population of England and Wales.

Life expectancy

Increases in life expectancy in industrialised countries

Life expectancy, along with infant mortality rate, is one of the most widely used measures of the health of populations. It is used to compare the health of different populations and for monitoring improvement (or deterioration) in health within a single population. Since the turn of the century, life expectancy at birth has increased very substantially in industrialised countries (e.g. from around 47 years in 1900 to around 75 years in both the UK and US; DH, 1992a; DHHS, 1992). Even if one corrects for the distorting effect of high infant mortality at the turn of the century by comparing life expectancies of one-year-olds, there has still been an increase in life expectancy of around 20 years over the course of this century. Life expectancy is still increasing in many industrialised countries; Figure 1.4 shows changes in life expectancy in four European countries since 1970. A very similar trend to that shown for European countries has also occurred in the USA over this period;

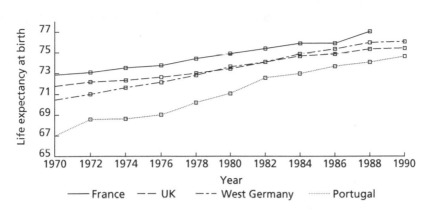

Figure 1.4 Life expectancy changes in four European countries 1970–1989. Data source: Echo (1993)

between 1970 and 1987 life expectancy increased from 72 to 75.6 years in white Americans and from 64 to 69.4 years in black Americans (DHHS, 1992). These dramatic increases in life expectancy, over the course of this century, have been largely achieved by reducing deaths, particularly deaths from infectious diseases, amongst children and younger adults. Deaths from infectious diseases like tuberculosis and other acute causes (e.g. deaths in childbirth) have declined very sharply over the last half century and now about three-quarters of all deaths are due to the chronic, age-related circulatory diseases and cancer.

Changes in life expectancy inevitably mean changing patterns of disease

In large measure, the great changes in the causes of morbidity and mortality in the USA and UK over this century have been an inevitable consequence of the increased life expectancy and of our success in preventing earlier deaths from other causes. If more people survive into old age, the diseases that become increasingly prevalent in old age must likewise become more prevalent. In the UK, circulatory diseases accounted for 26% of all deaths in 1931 but by 1991 this had risen to 46% of deaths, but over this same time period the proportion of deaths from many other causes, particularly infections, dropped very substantially (DH, 1992b). Portraying an increase in mortality resulting from cardiovascular diseases and cancer as a wholly negative phenomenon, as a modern epidemic that indicates the dangers of western diet and lifestyle, is somewhat misleading. If one reduces or eliminates deaths from some causes then it is inevitable that other causes must account for an increased proportion of the total. The present diet and lifestyle are not ideal and 'improvements' would almost certainly delay death and morbidity due to these chronic diseases, but the changes in diet and lifestyle that have occurred during this century have been accompanied by very large increases in life expectancy and improved health in 'western' industrial countries like the USA and UK.

In Japan these changes in mortality and morbidity patterns have been particularly rapid. Three classes of degenerative diseases – cancer, cardiovascular diseases and diabetes mellitus, now account for two-thirds of deaths whereas in 1950 they accounted for less than one-third of deaths. Crude death rates from cardiovascular disease and cancers have increased by around 250% since 1950. Yet Fujita (1992) suggests that when age-adjusted mortality rates are calculated and full allowance is made for the change in age distribution of the population over this period, the number of Japanese suffering from the chronic degenerative diseases has remained about constant over the last three decades. He concludes that the rise in crude mortality from heart disease and cancer is mainly due to increases in the actual number of elderly persons rather than, as is frequently suggested, due to the 'westernisation' of the Japanese diet. Life expectancy in Japan was approximately 49 years in 1935 but in 1991 was 79 years!

The elderly are also living longer now

Table 1.2 shows a comparison of life expectancy at different ages in the UK at the start of the century and in 1990. In absolute terms the differences in life expectancy between 1900 and 1990 get narrower as the starting age gets higher. Thus the difference between the two life expectancies at birth is around 29

Table 1.2 A comparison of approximate UK life expectancies at various ages in 1901 and 1991. Data source: DH (1992a)

| Age (in years) | Life expectancy (% compared) | | % increase |
	1901	1991	1901–1991
Birth	47	76	62
1	55	76	38
10	51	68	33
20	43	58	35
30	35	47	34
40	27	37	37
50	19	27	42
60	14	19	36
70	9	13	31
75	7.5	10.5	40

years whereas at the age of 60 years the difference is down to around 5 years. Nevertheless when expressed in percentage terms the increase in life expectancy after the first year remains relatively consistent right up to 70 years. The increased life expectancy of older people has generally been underestimated in the past. For example, projections of the number of over 85s there will be in 2001 are now 50% higher than the same projections made in 1974 (Grundy, 1992). Between the periods 1970–1972 and 1987–1989, the chances of a 65-year-old woman living a further 20 years increased from 33% to 44%. Not only are fewer younger people dying prematurely (i.e. before the age of 65 years) and surviving into old age but older people are also living much longer.

Increased life expectancy means more elderly people

The consequences of increased life expectancy, especially as in many countries it is coupled with low birth rates, means that there is an increasingly elderly population in many industrialised societies. Not only is the elderly population increasing in absolute terms but the elderly are also making up an increasing proportion of the total population. In the USA, the median age of the population is expected to rise from 29 years in 1975 to over 36 years by the turn of the century and by the end of the century 13% (35 million people) of

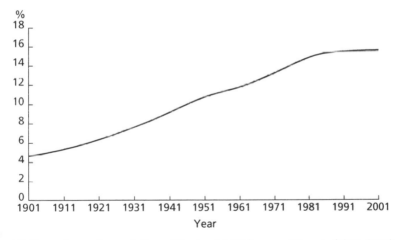

Figure 1.5 Percentage of population of England & Wales over 65 years (1901–2001). Data sources: Burr (1985); Grundy (1992)

the population in the USA are likely to be over 65 years with 2% of the population over 85 years (DHHS, 1992). Figure 1.5 shows changes in the proportion of elderly people in the UK population over the course of this century; the over 65s will have grown from less than 5% of the population at the turn of the century to almost 16% by the end of the century. By then the very elderly (over 85s) will number over 1 million and represent 2% of the population (from just over half a million in 1981). Longer term projections indicate that the number of people aged over 65 years in the UK will increase by 30% over the next 35 years and those over 85 years by 66% (DH, 1992a).

This ageing of affluent populations has important social, medical and economic implications.

Can these increases in life expectancy continue?

If one assumes that there are absolute genetic limitations to the life span of any particular person then increases in population life expectancy, like those described above, must have finite limits. Unless we can understand and control the ageing process and thus increase the life span, there must be limits to the extent that life expectancies can continue to rise. We may already be getting close to these limits in some industrialised countries. In Figure 1.6, survival curves for the UK in 1975, 1901 and British India 1921–1930 are compared; the shape of these curves is very different. At 60 years of age there are only around 10% survivors in the British India curve, just over half survive in the UK 1901 curve but around 85% in the UK 1975 curve. Despite this, the maximum age in these three graphs is about the same and the maximum human lifespan seems to be approximately 100–110 years. In Table 1.1, earlier in the chapter, there is evidence of a very rapid decline in the numbers of

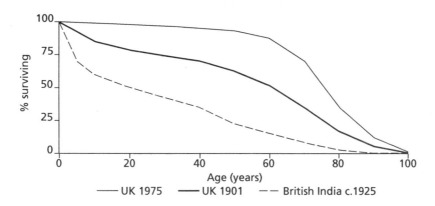

Figure 1.6 Survival curves for three human populations. Data source: Green (1994)

survivors at the extreme end of the age range; the 85–89 year age band represents 1.2% of the population but the whole of the 90+ age band, representing a potential 20+ year span, amounts to less than 0.5% of the population.

Improvements in public health, nutrition and medicine have allowed more people to survive for a longer proportion of their potential genetic life span; reduced mortality from the infectious diseases has been an important reason for this reduction in premature death. Much of health education and nutrition education these days is focused not upon infectious diseases and deficiency diseases but upon the chronic diseases of industrialisation which disable and kill principally middle-aged and older people. Diet and nutrition are considered to be significant factors in the aetiology of many of these chronic diseases that afflict elderly affluent populations. Eight of the top 11 causes of death in the USA are diet-related or alcohol-related conditions. The ultimate justification for almost all of adult nutrition education guidelines is the belief that if implemented they would delay the onset of cancers, diabetes mellitus and/or the cardiovascular diseases.

Life expectancy vs. expectations of life

Improving the total quality of life, rather than simply extending the duration of life, is now assuming an increasing priority as a health promotion objective. One of the major goals in *Healthy people 2000* in the USA (DHHS, 1992) is to 'increase the span of healthy life for Americans'. In the equivalent document in England, *The health of the nation* (DH, 1992b) the stated goal of the government is not only to reduce premature deaths and 'add years to life' but also to 'add life to years' by increasing the years that are free from ill-health and minimising the adverse effects of illness and disability. The emphasis is gradually shifting from extending the duration of life to reducing the impact of morbidity and disability in the later years of life and thus 'maintaining physical, emotional and intellectual vigour until shortly before death' (Katz *et al.*, 1983). (Note that there are Scottish and Welsh equivalents to *The health of the nation* which are similar in their broad aims and objectives to the English document.)

It was shown earlier in the chapter that the rate of disability increases roughly exponentially throughout adult life (Figure 1.3). This means that unless there are improvements in the health and general wellbeing of older people then increased life expectancy will be a flawed and imperfect measure of health improvement of populations. The optimistic view of future trends is that improved healthcare will, in the long term, continue to reduce morbidity and disability but will have a gradually diminishing effect upon life expectancy and so it will eventually tend to compress chronic morbidity and disability into a shorter period prior to death. The pessimistic view is that further increases in life expectancy will not be accompanied by corresponding improvements in morbidity leading to a large increase in the numbers of elderly people suffering from the chronic mental and physical disorders and disabilities that become more prevalent with age (Bebbington, 1988). For example, the prevalence of dementia increases markedly with age; the prevalence of Alzheimer's disease, the most common form of dementia, may increase 20-fold between the ages of 60 and 80 years. Moderate or severe dementia was found in 5–7% of over 65s in the UK and there are up to two million people in the EU with severe dementia (DH, 1991; and Echo, 1993). Likewise, the risk of osteoporotic fracture increases with age and affects mainly women, the bulk of the very elderly population. Unless the age-specific prevalence of dementia and osteoporosis can be reduced, then more elderly people inevitably means more people physically or mentally crippled by these conditions. At least for osteoporosis, the age-specific incidence of osteoporotic fracture seems to be increasing rather than decreasing in the UK (Spector *et al.*, 1990).

Years of life can be readily and reliably measured from the ages recorded on death certificates, but trying to assess the proportion of those total years that have been healthy, active years is much more difficult and inevitably going to be less precise. Katz *et al.* (1983) suggested 'active life expectancy' as an alternative to simple life expectancy as a measure of population health. They took as their end point for this measure not death, but the loss of independence in the activities of daily living, i.e. in bathing, dressing, eating and transfer (from bed to chair) which they determined by interview. Bebbington (1988) describes a method of calculating the 'expectation of life without disability' (ELWD). The ELWD is calculated from self-reported rates of disability and long-standing illness recorded in the British *General Household Survey* together with estimates of the numbers of people living in institutions for the 'disabled' (residential and nursing homes for the elderly, geriatric hospital wards and all forms of residential accommodation for the younger mentally and physically 'disabled').

Bebbington's method of calculating ELWD suggests that although total life expectancy in the UK increased over the period 1976–1988 ($\male$ from 70 to 72.4 years and $\female$ from 76.1 to 78.1 years) the years of active life remained essentially unchanged, because over this same period the years of illness and disability increased by 2.1 years in men and 2.5 years in women (DH, 1991). The main effect of the recent increases in life expectancy has been to increase the number of years spent suffering from illness and disability, that is to increase the dysfunctional period rather than the period of healthy life. A similar study in the USA (Crimmins *et al.*, 1989) concluded that between 1970 and 1980 increases in life expectancy were largely concentrated in years with a chronic disabling illness. Although the trend in ELWD is upward, it is rising more slowly than the increase in life expectancy and so the number of years that people spend suffering from chronic illnesses and disabilities is rising.

As might be expected, Bebbington found that elderly people have the worst outlook for ELWD. At birth, it is calculated that around four-fifths of the life expectancy will be without disability; however the proportion of the life expectancy that is predicted to be disability-free (the ELWD) falls rapidly in later adult life and is down to just over half by the age of 65 years. On a more optimistic note, Bebbington found that the greatest improvement in ELWD in England and Wales, over the period 1976–1985, was in the elderly age groups.

Changes in mortality causes with age

Table 1.3 shows that there are some very significant differences in the proportions of deaths accounted for by different causes in different age groups. Accidents, suicides and other violent deaths (injury and poisoning) account for almost two-fifths of deaths in young adults but considerably less than 2% of deaths in older adults. In young adults, heart disease accounts for 11% of all deaths, but rises steeply in middle age and accounts for about a third of deaths in the elderly. Cancer accounts for a quarter of all deaths in young

Table 1.3 Causes of death in different age groups in England and Wales. Data source: OPCS (1991)

Cause	Age group (years)					
	15–44	45–54	55–64	65–74	75–84	85+
Total deaths (000s)	19.6	21.7	58.9	131.4	198.0	127.6
% of deaths attributable to:						
Heart disease	11.0	27.7	32.9	34.1	32.4	28.9
Cancer	24.1	41.2	40.2	33.4	22.7	12.7
Cerebrovascular disease	3.3	5.1	5.8	9.0	14.4	16.7
Respiratory diseases	3.8	4.1	6.3	8.8	11.2	16.8
Injury and poisoning	38.0	8.3	2.9	1.5	1.3	1.3
Others	18.8	13.6	11.9	13.2	18.0	23.6

adults and more than 40% of deaths in middle age but then declines throughout old age so that in the over 85s it is responsible for only about one in eight deaths. Both cerebrovascular disease and respiratory diseases account for a steadily increasing proportion of deaths in older age groups. One must exercise some caution in interpreting such figures because of the reduced accuracy of certification of causes of death in older people. Pneumonia is, for example, frequently cited as the underlying cause of death in the very elderly and may partly account for the high proportion of deaths due to respiratory disease in the over 85s. Muscle weakness and reduced immunocompetence would both increase susceptibility to pneumonia and chest infections; both of these predisposing factors are associated with ageing and with malnutrition.

In young and middle-aged adults, there are very significant differences between the sexes in the relative importance of the major causes of mortality. In younger people, cancer and cerebrovascular disease account for a higher proportion of deaths in women than in men and the reverse is true for heart disease and accidents. In older adults, these differences narrow and the relative importance of the main causes of death is similar in the two sexes (see Table 1.4).

Causes of morbidity in the elderly

Earlier it was seen that rates of disability in all categories of severity rise with age; likewise, the proportion of people suffering from some longstanding illness also rises with age. In 1988, more than half of elderly people in Britain reported that they were affected by some longstanding illness; this proportion rises with age and is higher in women than in men (DH, 1992a). Despite this,

Table 1.4 Sex differences in the proportion of deaths attributed to various causes in the middle-aged and elderly. Data source: DH (1992a)

Cause	Age group (years)			
	55–64	65–74	75–84	85+
Men (000s)	34.9	77.2	95.8	39.3
Women (000s)	21.3	54.2	103.3	95.7
% of deaths attributable to:				
Circulatory diseases				
Men	47.0	48.0	49.0	46.0
Women	31.0	43.0	53.0	51 0
Neoplasms				
Men	36.0	33.0	25.0	17.0
Women	49.0	35.0	21.0	11.0
Respiratory system				
Men	6.0	9.0	13.0	20.0
Women	7.0	9.0	10.0	16.0
Other				
Men	11.0	9.0	13.0	18.0
Women	13.0	13.0	17.0	21.0

only a small percentage of the elderly people in Figure 1.2 reported that their health was bad; it seems that perhaps some level of disability and chronic disease may be seen as inevitable in old age and may not prevent people viewing their overall health as satisfactory or even good. Bone and joint diseases including arthritis and rheumatism are very common causes of long standing illness in the elderly, together with heart disease, hypertension, respiratory diseases (e.g. bronchitis and emphysema), stroke and diabetes (DH, 1992a).

Table 1.5 shows a breakdown of the reasons for general practitioner consultations by elderly people in England and Wales. This may give a fairly objective idea of the relative contribution of different categories of disease to the morbidity of older people. Diseases of the circulatory system, respiratory system and musculoskeletal system are the largest defined categories of diseases. When taking the population as a whole then the rate of consultation for most broad categories of disease increases with age. The effect of age on the consultation rate for individual diseases is more variable. In some cases, e.g. congestive cardiac failure, osteoarthritis, parkinsonism, cataract and varicose ulcers, there is a very marked increase in consultation rate with age. For some other conditions there is actually a decrease in consultation rate with age, for example upper respiratory tract infections, migraine and anxiety disorders.

Table 1.5 Percentage of elderly people in England and Wales consulting their general practitioner each year for various categories of conditions. Data source: DH (1992a)

% of elderly population	Condition category
over 25%	Circulatory diseases
20–25%	Musculoskeletal conditions Respiratory diseases Symptoms, signs and ill-defined conditions
10–20%	Diseases of the nervous system Mental disorders Diseases of the digestive system Injury and poisoning Diseases of the skin and subcutaneous tissues
5–10%	Diseases of the genitourinary system Infectious and parasitic diseases Endocrine, nutritional and metabolic diseases and immunity disorders
<5%	Neoplasms

High levels of long standing illness may increase the likelihood of malnutrition in the elderly. In the most recent surveys of the nutritional status of elderly people in the UK (DHSS, 1972 and 1979) malnutrition was usually associated with some predisposing medical or social condition. There is a general consensus that medical and social factors are key determinants of the nutritional status of elderly people.

In line with their high rate of general practitioner consultation, elderly people have much higher usage of prescribed and over the counter medications than younger people. Many older people take multiple medications on a daily basis. The need to consider possible drug-nutrient interactions is particularly relevant to those prescribing or catering for elderly people – this is discussed further in Chapter 5. In Chapter 8 there is some discussion of the role of diet in the management of certain diseases that are very common in the elderly.

Some characteristics of the elderly population in the UK

SEX RATIO

In young and middle aged adults, there are approximately equal numbers of men and women in the population of England and Wales, but as one progresses through the age bands of the over 60s then there is a marked increase in the proportion that is female. This dominance of females in the older age groups is expected to diminish only slightly by the end of the century (see Table 1.6). In the longer term, by 2026, the ratio of women to men in the over

Table 1.6 The proportion of females in various age bands of the UK population in 1991 with projections for 2001. Data source: Grundy (1992)

Age group	Year	% Female
65–74	1991	56
	2001	53
75–84	1991	63
	2001	60
85+	1991	75
	2001	73

85 age group is expected to fall from 3:1 to only 2:1 (DH, 1992a) as the gap between the life expectancy of men and women narrows.

Katz *et al.* (1983) in the US and Bebbington (1988) in the UK, both calculate that elderly men can expect a greater proportion of their remaining years to be disability-free than elderly women. According to Bebbington, at 65 years, the difference in the life expectancy of men and women was 3.5 years but the difference in the 'expectation of life without disability' was only 0.4 years.

In DH (1992a), it was also concluded that for most tasks, at all ages, the proportion of women reporting that they were unable to do the tasks independently was higher than the proportion of men. One explanation offered was that people living alone may be more aware of their limitations and more women live alone.

ETHNIC MIX

Most of the immigration to the UK from Asia and the Caribbean has occurred since the 1950s and most of the immigrants were relatively young when they arrived. This means that the ethnic mix of the elderly UK population is rather different from that of younger age groups. Only around 6% of the Afro-Caribbean and 2–3% of the Asian population in the UK in 1987–1989 were of pensionable age compared with 19% of the white population. The population of elderly people from the ethnic minorities in the UK is expected to increase rapidly over the next couple of decades (DH, 1992a).

Some economic implications of our ageing population

As the population ages and the elderly become an increasing proportion of the total population, so the number of people of working age declines as a proportion of the total. The 'aged dependency ratio' is the population aged

Table 1.7 Aged dependency ratios; the population over 65 years expressed as a percentage of the population of working age i.e. 15–64 years in four industrialised countries with projections to 2030. Data source: DH (1992a)

Country	Year		
	1990	2010	2030
West Germany (before unification)	22.3	30.6	43.6
USA	18.5	18.8	31.7
Japan	16.2	29.5	31.9
UK	23.0	22.3	31.1

65+ years as a percentage of the population of working age (15–64 years). Table 1.7 shows current aged dependency ratios in several industrialised countries and the projected changes in this ratio over the next 40 years.

Figure 1.7 shows a comparison of the sources of income of younger and older adults in the UK and illustrates the importance of projected rises in the aged dependency ratio. As would be expected, most of the income of the younger adults is 'earned' from employment or self employment, whereas most of the income of older people is from 'unearned' sources, much of it from the social security budget and occupational pension schemes. Much of this supply of 'unearned' income must come from the current contributions of younger, employed people.

In the medium term, the UK and US will see little change in this ratio, although major increases are projected in some countries such as Japan and Germany. In the longer term, this ratio will increase very substantially in

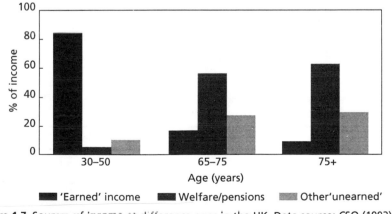

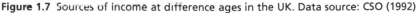

Figure 1.7 Sources of income at difference ages in the UK. Data source: CSO (1992)

almost all industrialised countries. This is the 'demographic time bomb' that is so frequently discussed in the media. It has, for instance, prompted discussion about the feasibility of maintaining the real value of the universal state pension in the UK. It is also curtailing the state financing of long term residential care for elderly people with disabilities.

In 1989/90, public expenditure upon health and social services for elderly people in England represented almost half of the total expenditure on these services (Robins and Wittenberg, 1992). Almost a third of this £11.3 bn ($17 bn) spent on health and social services for the elderly was spent on the 4% of elderly people receiving some form of publicly funded residential care. Over the 1980s, real expenditure on health and social services for the elderly rose at an annual rate of 3.4% per annum. Demographic trends, increasing utilisation rates for services and increased unit costs mean that this budget will need to continue rising at a real rate of at least 3% per annum. Any changes in the amount of informal care provided by relatives and friends could dramatically alter this projection. At present, substantially more hours of care are provided by informal carers than by formal sources. The cost of replacing this informal care has been estimated at as much as double the current total health and social services budget (Robins and Wittenberg, 1992).

Living circumstances of elderly people

As people get older, then the likelihood of their being able to manage household tasks and to be capable of living independently is reduced. This means that increasing numbers of very elderly people must be supported by living with younger relatives or be cared for in residential homes for the elderly.

In the UK, the proportion of elderly people living with their younger relatives has declined very substantially over the last few decades; Table 1.8 illustrates this decline in the extended family unit since the 1960s. More than four-fifths of the non-institutionalised over 65s now either live alone or with their spouse only, whereas in 1962 the corresponding figure was only just over half. The likelihood of older adults living alone increases sharply with age, largely due to the deaths of spouses. In the 65–69 year age group, about 15% of men and 30% of women live alone but in the 85+ year age group this rises to about 60% of women and 50% of men.

Table 1.8 Household circumstances of elderly people (over 65s) living in private households in the UK. Data source: DH (1992a)

	1962	1980	1989
Alone	22	34	36
With spouse only	33	45	46
With others	44	21	18

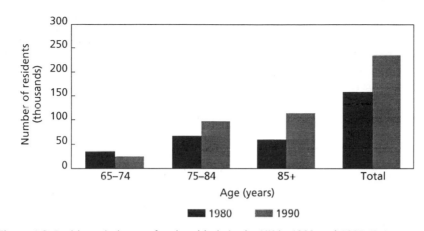

Figure 1.8 Residents in homes for the elderly in the UK in 1980 and 1990. Data source: DH (1992a)

The 1981 census showed that about 8% of the total population of Great Britain aged over 75 years lived outside private households, most of them in some sort of institution providing care. Partly because of the decline in the extended family, there has been a very substantial increase in the absolute numbers of people living in residential homes for the elderly (see Figure 1.8). In 1980 there were around 157,000 people aged 65+ years living in such residential homes and by 1990 this figure had grown to 235,000. This is a very obvious cost of an ageing population. The probability of living in a residential home for the elderly increases with increasing age; in 1990, around a half per cent of those 65–74 years, around 3.5% of those aged 75–84 years, but over 14% of those aged 85+ years (DH, 1992a). According to CWT (1995), if all types of long term care are included (i.e. residential homes, nursing homes and long stay hospitals) then the total proportions of the elderly living in care accommodation is as shown below:

- 1% of 65–74 year olds
- 5.9% of 75–84 year olds
- 26.6% of those aged 85+ years.

Although the absolute numbers have risen, the proportion of the elderly population that is in care accommodation has remained relatively stable. The increases illustrated in Figure 1.8 are largely explained by increases in the total numbers of elderly people. Younger elderly people are probably healthier and more independent than in the past, because the proportion of people aged 65–74 years living in residential homes actually declined during the 1980s, despite the reduced numbers living in extended families. The stated aim of the UK government in the Community Care Act 1993 is to enable people to stay in their own homes for as long as possible. This would be expected to reduce the proportion of elderly people living in care accommodation. Nevertheless, the projected rapid growth in the very elderly population, and the marked and longstanding tendency for less elderly people to live with their children, means that the numbers of people being cared for in residential homes for the elderly is unlikely to fall significantly and in the longer term is probably set to carry on rising. This not only has economic implications but also points to an increase in the numbers of people employed in caring occupations who will need to be educated about the care and needs of the elderly, including their nutritional needs.

Provision of residential care accommodation for the elderly

The growth in places for elderly people in nursing homes and residential homes over the last 20 years has been in private sector accommodation. Over the period 1977–1990, the number of residents in voluntary and local authority homes fell slightly, whereas the number of places in private residential homes increased from less than 25,000 places to around 120,000 places (DH, 1992a). The private sector now accounts for over half of all residential home places and the UK residential care home business had an estimated annual turnover of £4.5 billion ($6.7 billion) in 1993 (CWT, 1995).

Profitability is a proper and essential requirement for any private business. In this case, that business is the provision of care for vulnerable people who have a high prevalence of mental and physical disability and frailty. This emphasises the need for vigilance upon the part of all involved – regulatory and licensing authorities, relatives and friends of elderly people, and the staff and management of the homes themselves – to ensure that the need for profitability does not prevent the provision of good standards of food and other care. An expert group sponsored by the Caroline Walker Trust (CWT, 1995) estimated that in 1994 expenditure upon food ingredients in the various categories of residential homes (local authority, voluntary and private) varied from £11–21.50 per person per week ($16.50–32 pppw). Cost per head and nutritional content are not absolutely tied and some of this variation will be due to differences in the size of homes (in larger homes, and especially in those with local authority central spending power, economies of scale would be expected to lower per capita costs). Nevertheless, this expert group (CWT, 1995) considered that it would be difficult to provide adequate nutritional content for a weekly per capita expenditure of less than £15 ($22.50), 35% more than the estimated expenditure of some homes.

Social isolation in the elderly

As friends and relatives die or move away, then social isolation would be expected to increase with age in the elderly. A 1985 UK survey of elderly people living outside institutions, found only limited evidence of this increase in isolation with age. Only around 2% of those aged 65–69 years reported not seeing friends and relatives at all and around 85% reported seeing them at least once a week. In the over 85s, those not seeing friends and relatives at all had still only risen to about 4% and three-quarters of them were still seeing them at least once a week. However, these figures almost certainly underestimate the true rate of decline in the amount of time many people spend in social situations as they age. There is loss of the external contact through work, and reduced mobility may reduce participation in many leisure time pursuits, social visiting and even visits to shops. In the over 85s, around 30% of men and 50% of women are either permanently housebound or can only go out if helped (DH 1992a). Elderly people from ethnic minorities may well be further disadvantaged by their poor language skills unless they are supported by the traditional extended family.

In elderly people living in Gothenburg Sweden, loneliness was found to be a problem for 24% of women and 12% of men. The most important factors contributing to this loneliness were loss of spouse, depression of mood and lack of friends; living conditions sometimes increased the social isolation of elderly people. Living alone, poor vision and urinary incontinence were also common contributors to the social isolation of these elderly Swedes. These lonely elderly people had a generally negative view of their own health and were more demanding of medical and social care despite the lack of any higher prevalence of definable somatic disease (Steen, 1992).

Community centres, lunch clubs and visiting initiatives for the elderly can all make some contribution to reducing loneliness of the elderly. In areas with significant ethnic minority populations then these services will need to make provision for elderly people from minority communities, e.g. by providing culturally acceptable meals and by making provision for those with limited written or spoken English. Addressing practical problems like urinary incontinence, visual, hearing and mobility difficulties is also likely to reduce the likelihood of social isolation and loneliness. Given the Swedish findings above, there is likely to be a financial return in the form of reduced dependence upon medical and social services if loneliness amongst the elderly can be reduced.

Economic circumstances of elderly people

The household income and expenditure of elderly people in the UK tends to be concentrated at the lower end of the range. In both single adult and one man, one woman households, retired persons account for 40–80% of the three lowest household income groups but they become progressively less well represented in the higher income categories. Retired persons in the upper income groups inevitably receive some income in addition to the state pension. Figure 1.9 illustrates how age affects the household income in the UK. In 1992, over 60% of the households with an elderly head had an income of less than £175 ($260) per week compared to only about 15% of young adult households; less than 20% of older households have an income of over £325 ($485) per week compared to about 60% of young adult households. Within this large elderly age band, income declines with increasing age. Of course, Figure 1.9 gives a slightly distorted view of the per capita spending power of older households

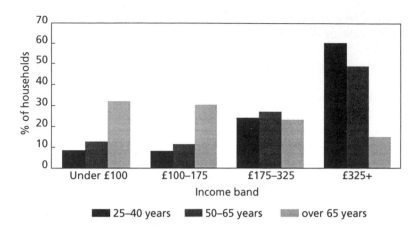

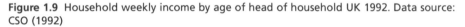

Figure 1.9 Household weekly income by age of head of household UK 1992. Data source: CSO (1992)

because the size of households will tend to be smaller in the older age brackets. Nevertheless, the average expenditure per person in households where the head was aged over 75 years, was only two-thirds of that in households where the head was aged 50–64 years. Old age is widely and, for many it would seem, correctly perceived as a time of relative poverty. The increasing ratio of retired to working people in the population and the increasing numbers living in costly, residential homes for the elderly, makes it difficult to foresee any marked improvement in the economic status of the bulk of elderly people in the UK unless this issue acquires a higher political priority.

Table 1.9 Food expenditure of one woman, one man households in the UK (£1 is approximately $1.5). Data source: CSO (1992)

	Food spending	
Household category	**£**	**% total spending**
Retired mainly dependent on state pension:		
Income <£120 pw	30.4	27.8
Income >£120 pw	35.5	22.6
Retired with additional income:		
Income <£200 pw	35.0	21.9
Income >£275 pw	47.3	15.2
Not retired:		
Income <£250 pw	39.0	20.2
Income £350–475 pw	47.0	16.7
Income >£650 pw	63.3	13.2

As income declines so expenditure also inevitably tends to decline and the proportion of total expenditure devoted to various commodities and services also changes. In general as income declines, so absolute per capita expenditure on food declines, but food accounts for an increasing share of the total expenditure (see Table 1.9). The proportion of income spent upon housing, fuel and food increases with age in Britain but the proportion spent on clothing, transport, alcohol and tobacco declines. Table 1.9 suggests that in 1992, retired couples in the lowest income group spent about £15 ($23) per person per week on food.

Food expenditure of older adults

The UK National Food Survey (NFS) is an annual record of one week's household food purchases of a representative sample of 7000–8000 households. This survey is an invaluable source of information about time trends in food purchasing practices in the UK and gives good information about regional variations in diet. It can also be used to identify differences between the food purchasing practices of different socioeconomic groups. One of the types of household identified in this survey is old age pensioners (OAP) – a household in which at least three-quarters of the total income comes from pensions or similar allowances and in which at least one member of the household is over the state retirement age. There are a number of problems about using the NFS to identify dietary differences between groups. These are listed below and should be borne in mind whenever interpreting information in this book that has been derived from the National Food Survey.

- It is an expenditure survey not a consumption survey; it measures the amount of food brought into the household during a particular period, not the amount consumed during that time. There is evidence that people, especially in the lower income groups, buy more food than usual during the survey week (see Leather, 1992). Different preparation practices (e.g. trimming of meat), differing levels of wastage, and changes in household food stocks during the survey period are just some of the factors that reduce its usefulness as a measure of food intake. The survey gives no indication of food distribution within the household.
- As households get larger, then per capita expenditure upon food tends to decline. This partly reflects economies of scale and partly reflects the fact that larger households usually contain children who eat less than adults. Most OAP households are composed of either single adults or couples. In this book, the expenditure patterns of OAP households have therefore usually been compared to those of single adult and two adult households. These two categories will include most OAP households (average number of persons per OAP household is 1.45) but the OAPs will make up only about 20% of the total. On a purely household composition basis, one might expect the expenditure of OAPs to lie somewhere between that of one and two adult households.

- The NFS does not record details of food purchased for consumption outside of the household. It records only the number of external meals eaten each week. In general, OAPs and lower income groups tend to eat fewer meals outside of the household than more affluent groups. Thus, in the 1992 survey (MAFF, 1993) 'two adult' households took an average of 2.5 meals per person per week (pppw) from outside the household supply, whereas the equivalent for OAP couples was only 0.9 pppw. There was a general decline in the number of external meals taken as the age of the main diary keeper in the household rose.
- The sample of OAPs in the NFS is not wholly representative of older people. It obviously excludes those living in care accommodation but more importantly, the poorest and frailest of the independent elderly are probably underrepresented in the sample (see Leather, 1992).

Table 1.10 shows a comparison of food expenditure by OAP households and by all single adult and two adult households. This confirms the finding in Table 1.9, that the per capita food expenditure of OAP households is less than that of other equivalent sized households; these data indicate that it is at least 12% less. The real gap is even higher than this because OAPs take fewer external meals and thus household food represents a higher proportion of total food expenditure than that of the other households. OAPs get substantially more calories per penny than either of the comparison groups; it is a general finding of the National Food Survey that as income and expenditure decline so the amount spent on each calorie of food energy declines, i.e. that poorer people buy cheaper foods. Expenditure upon soft drinks, alcoholic drinks and to a lesser extent confectionery was also lower in OAP households, with alcohol expenditure well under half that of the other two groups.

Is food spending by OAPs sufficient to purchase an adequate and healthy diet? In 1991, the UK Ministry of Agriculture, Fisheries and Food (MAFF) produced a 'low-cost, healthy diet' that could be purchased for £10 ($15) per person per week at 1991 prices. Using this £10 figure as a yardstick then the food expenditure of OAPs indicated by Tables 1.9 and 1.10 looks more than sufficient to enable even those reliant wholly on the state pension to purchase an adequate and healthy diet. However, it has been suggested that this £10 diet is so far removed from the normal eating pattern of the British population as to be totally unrealistic. The £10 diet would require, for example: almost total exclusion of meat and most dairy products from the diet; a very large increase in bread consumption and most of this bread would have to be eaten dry without butter or margarine; and large increases in consumption of tinned fruit and frozen vegetables (Leather, 1992). It is easy to produce lists of ingredients that meet any set compositional criteria within a very small budget but it is much more expensive to purchase a collection of ingredients that can also be combined into meals that make up a culturally acceptable diet. The Family Budget Unit at York University estimated the cost of a 'modest but adequate' diet which would not only be adequate and comply with current nutrition education guidelines but also be broadly in line with the usual diet of the UK population (see Leather, 1992). Using these criteria the minimum food expenditure of an adult couple

Table 1.10 Selective comparison of expenditure upon household food and drink of one adult, two adult, and OAP households from the UK National Food Survey (MAFF, 1993). Unless otherwise stated, values are pence per person per week (£1 or 100 pence is approximately $1.5)

Food	Household composition		
	1 adult	2 adult	OAP
Milk and cream	165	154	157
% low fat milk	34%	39%	31%
Cheese	56	55	42
Meat & meat products	373	424	352
Fish & products	99	100	92
Eggs	27	23	26
Fats	47	47	51
Sugars and preserves	27	24	33
Vegetables	201	215	149
% potatoes	13%	14%	20%
Fruit	142	137	114
Cereals	261	247	222
Beverages	60	57	63
Total food spending	£15.3	£15.6	£13.6
Food (kcals per penny)	1.38	1.35	1.60
Soft drinks	37	37	24
% low calorie	23%	31%	14%
Alcoholic drinks	130	151	58
Confectionery	23	25	21
Total food and drink	£17.2	£17.8	£14.6

was around £17 per person per week at 1992 prices. Using this £17 figure then the food expenditure of the poorest OAPs looks to be much more borderline. Note that the above costings were based upon the nutritional requirements of younger adults, and older people may need slightly less food.

Are the food purchasing patterns of OAPs broadly similar to those of the comparison groups? Can we assume that the contribution of particular foods to the supply of key nutrients is similar in young and older adults?

The figures in Table 1.10 suggest that there are significant differences. The amounts spent upon cheese, vegetables (especially those other than potatoes) and fruit are all substantially lower in the OAP households; purchases of soft drinks and alcohol are also substantially lower. Of course, some differences in absolute expenditure are inevitable, given the lower total spending of OAP households. When the proportion of the total food expenditure that is spent upon various food groups is calculated then the above differences between the groups narrow and in some cases disappear. Thus OAPs and the comparison groups spend similar proportions of their food expenditure upon dairy food, meat and fish, and cereals; they still seem to spend less upon vegetables and perhaps fruit. OAPs spend more in absolute terms upon sugars and fats than the comparison groups despite the lower total expenditure. It is, of course, difficult to know how important economic constraints are as a direct cause of these differences between the food purchasing patterns of OAPs and the comparison groups.

It is interesting to note from Table 1.10 that the proportion of soft drink expenditure that is used to buy low calorie drinks is much lower in the OAP group, and that less of the milk bought by the OAPs is low fat milk. This is consistent with a tendency for older people to be more traditional in their food purchasing and to lag behind trends in the purchasing habits of the population in general. This point is discussed again in Chapter 2 where trends in fat purchases are analysed.

Food selection in elderly adults

Aims and introduction

The aim of this chapter is to overview the non-nutritional influences upon the food choices of elderly people. An understanding of the reasons for food choices, and identification of such key influences is essential for effective practical dietary advice whether it be for health promotion, ensuring adequacy or for the dietary management of disease. People seldom choose their food solely upon nutritional grounds or on the basis of chemical composition. Geographical, seasonal, economic, cultural and preference factors largely determine what people eat. For some people, (those living in institutions for example) food choices may be largely imposed upon the individual from outside. A prescribed diet or recommended dietary improvement may be ideal from the biological viewpoint but it will almost certainly be ineffective if it is, for example, culturally unacceptable, incompatible with the food offered by a caterer, incompatible with personal preferences or beliefs, or beyond the economic means of the individual. Food is only nutritious when it is actually eaten!

Some of the nutrition education tools used to aid people in diet selection (food groups, the Food Guide Pyramid and the Food Guide Plate) will also be described in this chapter and discussed in relation to their use with older people.

Finally, some of the barriers that hinder the implementation of nutrition or other health promotion advice and some factors that influence the likelihood of recommended dietary changes being implemented by elderly people will be discussed. These would be essential considerations for anyone hoping to design a successful nutrition education programme or health promotion campaign for elderly people.

Non-nutritional uses of food

Food fulfils numerous social, psychological and cultural roles in addition to its biological role of providing energy and nutrients. Some of these non nutritional uses of food are listed in Table 2.1 with some specific examples; it is not suggested that this list is definitive, it is merely intended to illustrate the great diversity of non-nutritional uses of food. The non-biological functions of food may be particularly important in those elderly people whose opportunities for socialising, participating in work, leisure and other pleasurable activities are limited. Radical changes to a person's diet may impair the capacity of food to fulfil its non-biological functions and consequently reducing the pleasure gained from food may amount to a major reduction in the quality of life of some elderly people. The general approach recommended when devising diets or nutrition education advice for the elderly, or indeed for any group, is the 'cultural conservationist' approach (Webb, 1995) which is to recommend changes that produce the maximum biological benefit for the minimum disruption to the chosen diet and lifestyle of the individual.

Those recommending dietary change have a duty to ensure that there are good grounds for believing that such changes will yield holistic benefits for the individual or population group targeted. It should not be assumed that dietary changes are innocuous and thus that even if recommended changes or prescribed diets do no good neither will they do any harm. There is a tendency to recommend dietary changes on flimsy, sometimes highly speculative grounds, because of the assumption that they are inevitably a 'one-way bet' and even if they fail to work no harm has been done. This is an illogical assumption; if dietary change can produce major differences in wellness, life expectancy or the symptoms of a disease then there must be the potential to do harm as well as good. It should be assumed that any change that does no good will probably do some harm; this may be direct physiological harm or more probably economic, social or cultural harm. Anyone who has followed a prescribed diet will know that this has a social and quality of life cost; continual awareness of the need to follow a diet (or change any behaviour for supposed health reasons) may foster a morbid preoccupation with illness and death. This issue is discussed at length in Webb (1995).

A food selection model

Explanation

Discussions about the myriad of influences upon the dietary practices of a group can end up being an amorphous and confusing jumble of ideas and facts. Table 2.2 lists a variety of factors that can affect food choices and eating patterns. Many authors have tried to organise and integrate these various and disparate influences upon food selection into a simple but comprehensive model of food selection. Webb (1995) has previously used the idea of a

Table 2.1 Some non-nutritional uses of food

Food use	Example
As a religious symbol or an accessory in religious ceremonies and rituals	Use of bread and wine in Christian communion to symbolise the body and blood of Christ
To demonstrate piety or the distinctiveness of a religious group	Adherence to the strict dietary rules of the Torah by orthodox Jews
To make a moral or political statement	Past boycotts of foods from South Africa or avoidance of meat because of animal welfare concerns
To show esteem To demonstrate one's wealth and success	Serving expensive and/or elaborately prepared food to guests
Initiate or maintain a personal relationship	Inviting a new neighbour or acquaintance to a meal
To demonstrate/differentiate social status	Use of different dining facilities by different grades of employees
To demonstrate religious authority	Severe penalties for alcohol consumption in some Moslem countries
To exercise political power	Subsidising or rationing of foods Use of food aid as a political lever
As a punishment or reward	Traditional bread and water punishment for prisoners Sweets/candies as a reward for children
As a therapy in folk medicine	In the traditional Chinese system, foods classified as 'hot' may be used to treat a disease classified as 'cold'
To demonstrate love/caring	Gifts of food Care in preparation of food and/or feeding a sick person
To help forge and maintain family bonds	Sharing food in formal family meals

hierarchy of food availability to construct a model of food selection (see Figure 2.1). This model will be used later as a framework to discuss the particular influences upon the dietary practices of older people.

The basic concept of this hierarchy is that various factors affect the real availability of foods to the individual and thus the chances of foods being

Table 2.2 Some factors affecting food choice and eating patterns

Availability of foods in the local environment (in turn influenced by several factors like climate, soil type, transportation links, rationing, shopping facilities)

Nutrition knowledge and/or food beliefs (in turn influenced by such things as cultural traditions, education, religious/ethical beliefs)

Habit and previous food experience

Individual likes and dislikes

Facilities for storing, preparing and cooking

Cooking just for oneself or eating with and/or cooking for others

Skills in food preparation and willingness to experiment and develop new skills

Financial resources, budgeting skills and the cost of foods (these may be affected by political decisions about taxation, subsidy and welfare payments)

Time available and the time required to prepare and eat foods

State of health and appetite

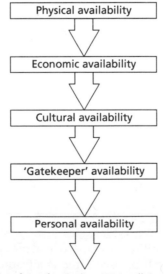

Selection from foods that are 'really' available

Figure 2.1 A model of food selection based upon the concept of a hierarchy of constraints upon food availability. Source: Webb (1995)

consumed. It is suggested that although, in theory, the affluent western consumer has almost total lack of restriction upon food choices, in practice there
are often very great practical limitations upon real freedom of choice. These
influences may range from absolute unavailability or sole availability to subtle increases or decreases in the availability. For example:

- changes in affordability can make a food absolutely unavailable, an occasional treat or an attractive cheap filler for those on low incomes
- the meal offered by a 'gatekeeper' (e.g. the caterer in a hospital or residential home) may be all that is available; the clients either eat it or go hungry
- advertising may increase the cultural, gatekeeper or personal availability of
  a food whereas negative health promotion messages may decrease it.

The practical limitations on availability may severely restrict the ability of
consumers to implement dietary guidelines or to follow prescribed diets
unless the advice has been framed with such limitations in mind. It is suggested that these influences upon availability can be arranged into a hierarchy
or series of hurdles; there must be at least a minimum availability at lower levels in the hierarchy before determinants of availability higher up in the
hierarchy become significant.

Origins of the food selection model

The model in Figure 2.1 is based upon an idea familiar to many psychologists,
Maslow's theory of motivation, which uses the concept of a hierarchy of
human needs (Maslow, 1943). Needs lower down this hierarchy must be at
least partially satisfied before the needs higher up the hierarchy become motivating (these are summarised in Figure 2.2). In Maslow's theory, the more
basic biological and emotional needs come at the start of the hierarchy, only
when there is reasonable satisfaction of these needs do the more aesthetic and
esoteric needs become significantly motivating.

Maslow's hierarchy – one reason for the differing dietary practices, beliefs and attitudes of young and old?

The elderly population in the UK will have been children before the age of
apparently limitless abundance and range of foods that has been with us
since the end of the 1950s. For many elderly people in the UK, their formative years will have been spent during the years of wartime shortages and
rationing. For elderly people from poor families, who were children before
the outbreak of World War II, their formative childhood experiences will
have been of parents struggling to provide an adequate diet; personal sacri-
fices by parents to ensure that the children were fed will often be an abiding
and dominating memory. Thus during the formative years of many elderly
people, the first three tiers of Maslow's hierarchy will have been the pre-
dominant motivating influences upon food selection. For most younger
adults whose childhoods have been spent during the years of plenty only the

Self-actualisation
At the pinnacle of the hierarchy of motivation is the need for self-actualisation – use of food choices to demonstrate one's individuality and uniqueness, e.g. serving food that demonstrates distant ethnic roots by someone who normally eats the diet of the majority of the population.

Self-esteem
Next, the need for self esteem becomes an important motivating influence. Food may be used as a means of demonstrating status and wealth.

Love-belongingness
When future security is relatively assured, then love-belongingness becomes a motivation priority. This could be manifested by the use of food to demonstrate love and caring or the use of food to demonstrate group membership.

Security
When there is no immediate threat to survival, future security becomes motivating – this may manifest as food storage or hoarding.

Survival
In extreme deprivation, survival is the sole motivating factor – people will usually eat almost anything that is remotely edible.

Figure 2.2 Maslow's theory of human motivation (after Maslow, 1943)

higher three tiers of Maslow's hierarchy will have been major motivating influences. Similarly, what little nutrition education elderly people would have experienced in their childhoods would have had nutritional adequacy as its sole aim, or at least its overriding priority. Over the last 35 years, the emphasis of nutrition education in industrialised countries has changed from ensuring adequacy to preventing the diseases of industrialisation like cancer, cardiovascular disease and maturity-onset diabetes. Nutrition education now emphasises moderation and restriction of many foods that were previously regarded as high prestige, luxury foods and in many cases viewed positively by nutrition educators as rich sources of essential nutrients and protein. Such foods include whole milk, cheese, eggs and meat. Many of the very elderly were children before any real scientific knowledge of essential nutrients and food composition existed, that is before the era of modern nutritional science and science-based nutrition education.

These differences in formative experiences may mean that the elderly have different attitudes to particular foods and different selection priorities to those of younger adults. Many of those giving dietary advice to the elderly have been brought up in the age of plenty and have never experienced food short-age or insecurity. They may find it difficult to understand food beliefs, habits and selection practices that have their origins in these earlier times of relative food scarcity, and which to them may seem irrational, even bizarre. Those seeking to influence the food selection of older adults would be well advised to seek to understand the origins of current beliefs and practices; 'dietary rec-ommendations that are devised with due regard to, and in sympathy with existing beliefs, preferences and selection practices will fare better than those that try to impose the prejudices and preferences of the adviser' (Webb, 1995).

The food selection model – influences upon availabilities in older adults

In this section, some of the array of factors that influence the food selection of older people are discussed using the food selection model in Figure 2.1 as the framework for the discussion. One point that must be re-emphasised is that although certain trends and changes may be associated with ageing, the elder-ly are a particularly heterogeneous group. It is undoubtedly true that elderly people are more likely than young adults to be disabled, immobile, poor and dependent. The following discussion and to some extent this book focuses upon these negative social, physiological and nutritional consequences of age-ing. Nevertheless, it should be remembered that even many very elderly people are healthy, active, reasonably affluent and have a very 'modern out-look'. For some people, retirement from work is associated with increased time and opportunity for engaging in leisure time pursuits, shopping and socialising; for them, the early retirement years may mean increased activity, mobility and socialisation rather than the decreases suggested by the general trends.

Physical availability

To be available and selected, the first requirement is for a food to be physical-ly available in the individual's environment. Seasonal and geographical factors are obvious examples of influences upon physical availability. In older people, reduced mobility could be a factor that limits the range of foods that are really available. There is an increasing tendency for shoppers to use large supermarkets that are located some distance from their homes, often on the outskirts of town. Small local shops have disappeared completely in some rural areas; where they remain, they tend to be relatively more expensive than large superstores and stock a narrower range of goods. A number of factors may reduce the mobility of older people and thus restrict their access to these larger stores or in some cases to shops in general:

- Low levels of cardiopulmonary fitness and strength (see Chapter 4). Even where this does not prevent travel, the ability to carry heavy loads may be limited and this may affect food choices or the amount that can be obtained during each shopping trip.

- The prevalence of disability increases with age; older people are more likely to suffer from a whole range of conditions that tend to reduce mobility, e.g. circulatory diseases like angina and intermittent claudication; musculoskeletal conditions like arthritis, gout and osteoporosis.
- Older adults are less likely than younger adults to have access to a car. Table 2.3 gives some estimates of car ownership in different categories of retired and non-retired households. Retired persons are less likely to have access to a car; only 8% of those living alone and largely on the state pension have access to a car. Within the retired categories rates of car ownership would drop with age.

As many as a third of UK men and half of women aged over 85 years and living at home are either completely housebound or can only go out with help. Lack of mobility may also affect the ability to prepare meals; more than a quarter of UK over 85s are unable to cook a main meal (DH 1992a). Reduced mobility and reduced access to a freezer (see Table 2.3) may compound to limit access to perishable foods or increase the likelihood of stale food being consumed; reduced taste and smell acuity may further increase the chances of stale or even spoiled food being consumed. Limitations on the availability of food preparation utensils or cooking facilities may also restrict the physical availability of food. For example, a baked potato can be prepared in a few minutes in a microwave oven. It can also be prepared in a conventional oven, but the time required and the fuel wasted to prepare a single potato may make this an impractical food for many single or widowed elderly people.

Table 2.3 Percentage of households owning consumer items by household type. Data source: CSO (1991)

Household type	Car	Fridge	Freezer
One adult			
Retired			
State pension	8	95	45
Other retired	37	98	68
Not retired	55	95	64
One man, one woman			
Retired			
State pension	46	99	71
Other retired	73	99	86
Not retired	88	99	92

'State pension' means living almost entirely upon the state pension, the 'other retired' have significant additional sources of income.

Over the period 1976–1987 the number of food shops in Britain fell by almost a third – the trend is very strongly towards a smaller number of larger retail outlets. This trend must inevitably mean that the average distance that consumers need travel in order to do their shopping has also increased. These new large retail outlets are increasingly located on the outskirts of towns where access is dependent upon use of cars or access to public transport; in 1988, two-thirds of new superstores were opened on the edge of towns and only about 10% in shopping centres or high streets. In line with this trend around 70% of households now make their shopping trips using a car. In order to take full advantage of these large superstores with their wide choice and low prices consumers need: good mobility (preferably access to a car), the financial resources to enable them to buy larger quantities and shop less frequently and good food storage facilities (including ownership of a freezer). In all of these respects the elderly, and especially the very elderly, are likely to be disadvantaged (statistics from Henson, 1992).

Economic availability

Some expensive foods, although available physically, may be economically unavailable to the poorer members of a community. Evidence has already been presented in Chapter 1 that elderly people are disproportionately represented in the lowest income groups in the UK. Per capita spending on food is lower in retired households than in comparably sized younger households and this is particularly so for those living largely upon the state pension. Food spending also accounts for a much greater proportion of total spending in these low-income elderly households (see Table 1.9). The question of whether the food expenditure of low-income, elderly people is sufficient to enable them to purchase a 'modest but adequate' diet was considered in Chapter 1.

A low income makes it difficult to live at maximum economic efficiency; often 'the poor pay more' and sometimes the elderly poor pay even more. Limited money, together with the small size of most elderly households may force the elderly to buy food in small expensive quantities; over 80% of elderly UK households consist of either one or two persons. Where elderly people have to buy larger quantities this may increase wastage or result in consumption of stale or spoiled food. Table 2.4 shows a rather anecdotal illustration of the potential magnitude of some of the differing costs of buying in small and large quantities. One of the authors (GW) surveyed the differences in unit cost of the same brands of common grocery items in a large London supermarket. The general trend was for decreasing unit cost with increasing pack size; there was often a sharp decrease in unit cost often between the smallest pack and the next smallest size, effectively penalising particularly the single person. Special offers tended to be concentrated in the largest packs and many special offers were in the form of discounts for multiple purchases. Clearly in the case of some goods (canned or heavily packaged foods) the non-food costs of the product are not much affected by the reduced size of the food portion and thus the differentials are inevitable.

For others, the marketing strategies of the retailer and producer work to the disadvantage of those like the single elderly, who need to buy in small quantities.

One would generally expect all household costs (e.g. replacement of capital items, rental charges and fuel costs) to rise on a per capita basis as the size of the household decreases, so increasing the pressure on the food budget of poor, small households. The elderly 'feel the cold' more than younger people

Table 2.4 Differences in costs of small and large packs of a variety of grocery items obtained from a large London supermarket in early 1995. All comparisons are between same brands and prices are pence per unit (variable) and so are directly comparable within items

Item	Small size	Unit price (pence)	Large size	Unit price (pence)	% price difference
Cucumber	half	70	whole	49	43
Mushrooms	1/4 lb	155	1 lb	115*	35
Peas (can)	142 g	8.3	300 g	5.4	54
Margarine	250 g	14.8	1 kg	11.9	24
Corned beef	198 g	36.4	340 g	28	30
Rice	500 g	11.8	4 kg	9.3	27
Baked beans	150 g	14	420 g	7.4	89
Chicken	1/4	99	whole	68*	46
Eggs	6	98	12	89	10
Oil	500 ml	74	1 l	59	25
Weetabix	12	68	48	46	48
Tea bags	40	40.8	160	33.8	21
Milk	1 pt	28	6 pt	22.2	26
Instant coffee	50 g	212	300 g	179	18
Washing up liquid	500 ml	126	1 l	99*	26
Sugar	500 g	90	1 kg	62	45
Burgers (frozen)	4	43.7	20	38	15
White bread	400 g	6	800 g	4.4	36
Flour	500 g	48	1.5 kg	27.4	75

* denotes special offer

and are more susceptible to hypothermia; poverty may force them to choose between adequate amounts of heating fuel or adequate food. The elderly poor are less likely to be able to stock up when a seasonal food is cheap or when special offers are made; only 45% of retired people who live alone and depend largely upon the state pension own a freezer (see Table 2.3).

As discussed above, the elderly may not have the transportation or personal mobility to enable them to shop at the most economic places. They may be forced to shop in smaller, more accessible but more expensive stores. These differences in costs between different retail outlets can be very substantial as a couple of examples illustrate. The unit cost of milk bought in half gallons from large supermarkets in the UK is only just over half of that from the traditional doorstep delivery services; in the spring and summer of 1994, several major supermarket chains were offering sliced white bread at around 40% of the cost in many small independent grocers. In a survey conducted in the Reading and Oxford areas of England in 1991, the cost of a basket of 21 food items was about a quarter higher in small independent grocery stores than in the supermarkets owned by the large multiple chains (Henson, 1992).

Decreased mobility and increased likelihood of disability may make it difficult for some elderly people to prepare cooked meals from raw ingredients. For those living alone, cooking just for themselves can considerably reduce the motivation to spend time and effort cooking. There is an enormous range of convenience and ready-prepared foods that would seem to offer a solution to this problem, although these are generally more expensive than the cost of the raw ingredients. Such convenience foods may nevertheless make an important contribution to maintaining a varied, palatable and nutritious diet for many older people. The practical costs of these convenience foods may sometimes be less than the real costs of buying minimum quantities of all of the ingredients, the costs of preparation and the costs of any wasted surplus ingredients. A can of vegetable soup may be more expensive than the cost of the raw ingredients but much cheaper than the real cost of preparing a small quantity of soup from raw ingredients. Factors such as this may change the balance of 'economic availabilities' for some foods between large families of younger people and older adults living alone or just with their spouses. For those unable to cook for themselves, relying largely upon cold foods also has its disadvantages: the diet is less varied and palatable, quite different from the diet of the culture and the minimum cost of eating a healthy diet is likely to be higher (perhaps around 15% higher according to Leather, 1992).

Cultural availability

Some foods may be physically and economically available but culturally unacceptable and thus unavailable to the consumer. This is most obvious in some of the strict and absolute religious prohibitions against the consumption of certain foods such as pork by Jews and beef by Hindus. There are also some foods that have great cultural significance which enhances their cultural availability. For example, rice is not only an important dietary staple in Japan but eating and cultivating rice is also important to many aspects of Japanese culture.

Jelliffe (1967) used the term 'cultural superfoods' to describe foods with major cultural, as well as nutritional, significance. Those giving dietary advice to people from a different ethnic background need to familiarise themselves with the 'food ideology' of their clients and to offer advice that is compatible with traditional beliefs and practices and with any religious dietary rules. This clearly applies whether the clients are young or old but the older members of a community are likely to be more fixed in their ways and less likely to accept changes that are inconsistent with traditional beliefs and practices.

The majority of the UK (or US) population does not follow a rigid and formal set of religious dietary rules. All cultures do, however, have less formal dietary conventions. Potentially edible materials are classified into food and non-food. Many of the plants, animals and insects in our environment are not eaten and not viewed by most Britons as food; cows, chickens, cabbages and crabs are seen as food but not horses, crows, nettles or frogs. There are also fairly fixed ideas about which foods are appropriate for particular meals, for particular occasions or for particular sections of the population. For example, cheese, salad vegetables, boiled vegetables and mashed potatoes are all part of many British diets but few Britons would consider these as potential breakfast foods; perhaps many would also put most fresh fruits in this category.

In the earlier discussion of Maslow's 'hierarchy of human needs', it was suggested that there were considerable differences in the range and abundance of foods and differences in nutritional priorities during the formative years of older people compared to more recent times. This may have caused subtle differences in the 'cultural availability' of some foods to young and old; attitudes to some foods may be very much affected by age. Nutrition educators and dietitians may be less sensitive to these more subtle cultural differences between young and old than they are to the more extreme and more obvious cultural differences between ethnic groups. The following examples illustrate how and why the images (cultural availability) of some foods may vary with age.

- There has been a major growth in the UK market for wholemeal bread over the last 10–15 years. This has been prompted by the current emphasis on dietary fibre in nutrition education and by improvements in the texture of wholemeal bread. In earlier years, the coarser brown and wholemeal breads were regarded as inferior to white bread and seen as the food of the poor or a few bran enthusiasts. 'Pure' white bread was seen as of higher prestige and palatability than bread made with less refined flour. In the period from World War II through to the mid-1950s, the manufacture of white bread was not allowed in the UK as an austerity measure. As soon as the restrictions on the manufacture of white bread were lifted in the mid 1950s, the sales of brown bread plummeted and white bread sales showed a corresponding sharp rise. The images of wholemeal bread may thus be completely different in young and old. The young, brought up in the fibre era, with a moist-textured wholemeal bread, may see it as the more natural, more flavourful and more wholesome product. The older adult may see it as a crude product, inferior in palatability and prestige to white bread.

- Attitudes to the different types of dietary cooking and 'spreading fats' may also be different amongst young and old. Before 1960 the UK market for vegetable oils, soft margarine and low-fat spreads was low or non-existent; butter and hard margarine were the usual spreading fats supplemented by lard and other animal-based fats for cooking. Table 2.5 shows how, even since 1975, there have been major shifts in the choice of cooking and spreading fats in the UK; vegetable oils, soft margarine and low-fat spreads have largely replaced the traditional cooking and spreading fats. Before the modern preoccupation with cholesterol and saturated fat, butter was generally regarded as the most palatable and natural of the 'yellow fats'; the hard margarine then available was regarded as a cheap, artificial and very inferior substitute to butter. In the period after the end of World War II, as supply problems and rationing were eased, then per capita butter consumption trebled in the UK. Since the concerns about saturated fat and cholesterol started being publicised in the 1960s and 1970s so per capita butter consumption has fallen sharply in the UK and is now below consumption during the period of imposed rationing in World War II (MAFF, 1993).

Table 2.5 A comparison of the relative popularity of different types of fat in the UK in 1975 and 1992. Data source: MAFF (1993)

'Yellow fats'	1975	1992
% butter	68	24
% soft margarine	14	43
% other margarine	18	3
% low fat spread	—	30
Other fats		
% oils	22	66
% lard type	69	22
% others	9	12

Figure 2.3 shows how the changing attitudes to different types of dietary fat have had a differential effect upon choice of fats amongst different age groups in the UK. There is a clear age-dependent decrease in the likelihood of choosing low-fat spread and a clear age-dependent increase for butter. As recently as 1975, butter formed a similar proportion of total fat purchases in all age groups except the over 75s (low fat spreads did not exist in 1975). There are also age-associated differences in the use of vegetable and salad oils; these account for a lower proportion of total fat purchases amongst the over 65s than they do in households with a younger diary keeper (MAFF, 1993).

Those giving dietary advice to older people or catering for older people cannot assume that they have the same attitudes to all foods as younger people; the 'cultural availability' of some foods may be very age dependent. A sandwich made with wholemeal bread and low fat spread may be viewed by many younger people as healthier, perhaps even more 'natural' than one made with white bread and butter. Older people are more likely to regard this option as of inferior quality, lower palatability and more unnatural. Such differences of image are likely to affect the acceptability of these two alternatives to young and old.

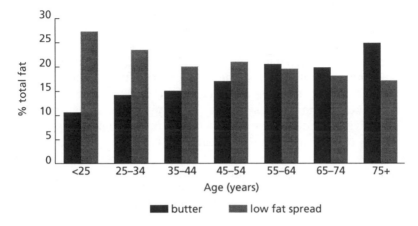

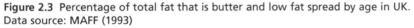

Figure 2.3 Percentage of total fat that is butter and low fat spread by age in UK. Data source: MAFF (1993)

Sizer and Whitney (1994) emphasise the importance of social interaction at meal-times which greatly enhances the pleasure of eating. In the widest sense, it helps to maintain or improve appetite and thus contributes to maintaining an adequate intake of essential nutrients. Many elderly people live alone and have little opportunity for social eating. Sizer and Whitney use an extended version of the following quotation to emphasise this point:

> [Preparing food] 'for one's self lacks the condiment of another's presence which can transform the simplest fare to the ceremonial act with all its shared meaning.'
> J. Weinberg (1972) Journal of the American Dietetic Association 60, 293–296.

The opportunity to take some meals with others may do more to maintain the nutritional status and quality of life of some older people than the provision of extra food for eating alone; relatives and neighbours concerned for the welfare of an older person are encouraged to consider this point. Access to lunch clubs or community centres where communal meals are served for older people is one way of attempting to address this issue.

Gatekeeper availability

The term 'gatekeeper' has been used to describe someone who controls the flow of food to others. It is most often used to describe the role of the mother in a traditional two parent family. The preferences and beliefs of the gatekeeper can impose severe limitations on choices available to other family members.

Old people living in residential care will have their meals provided by the caterer. There may be very restricted choices offered on the menu, especially in small institutions, and so the caterer's gatekeeping influence over the range of foods consumed by residents may be almost total. Low cost, ease of preparation and low need for staff involvement in serving and feeding clients are likely to be high on the caterer's list of priorities. The absolute numbers of older people living in residential homes for the elderly has been increasing rapidly over the last 20 years; more than a quarter of the over 85s live in some form of care accommodation. The diets of a large minority of elderly people are therefore very much in the hands of caterer-gatekeepers. This highlights the need for measures to improve the knowledge and understanding of these gatekeepers of the nutritional needs, priorities and potential nutritional problems of older people. The catering priorities above must not be allowed to prevent older clients being offered an appetizing and palatable diet in a convivial atmosphere. Those catering for the elderly need to be made aware of the importance of dietary adequacy in the elderly and encouraged to be more vigilant in seeking signs of poor nutrition and poor intake amongst their elderly clients.

Other gatekeeper influences that are likely to particularly affect the elderly are the meals provided by caterers for the 'at home' elderly such as community meals (e.g. meals delivered by 'meals on wheels') and those offered at community lunch clubs for the elderly. Catering standards for food in residential and nursing homes and for community meals are discussed in Chapter 7.

Until relatively recently, it has been traditional in most UK households for the wife/mother to act as the family gatekeeper; she has been largely responsible for planning, purchasing and preparing the family food. The loss of a gatekeeper spouse can leave many elderly men ill-equipped to cater for themselves. Conversely, the loss of a husband can leave some elderly women with little motivation to provide a varied and nutritious diet just for themselves (see the earlier quote from J. Weinberg). In the most recent national survey of the diets and nutritional status of older UK adults (DHSS, 1979) recent bereavement was one of the social factors associated with nutritional inadequacy.

Personal availability

At the end of the hierarchy a number of personal factors are left that can affect the availability of foods which have overcome all of the previous barriers to selection. Such factors include the following.

Personal preferences – a strong dislike of a food means that it is unlikely to be consumed no matter how favourable all of the other factors are.

Individual intolerance – adverse symptoms associated with a particular food, whether of physiological or psychological origin, mean that the food will be avoided.

Personal beliefs about foods – these may have considerable positive or negative influences irrespective of whether they have a rational basis or are based solely upon prejudice.

Below some individual factors that may alter the 'personal availability' of foods for older people are listed.

- Lack of teeth or ill-fitting dentures may reduce the consumption of foods that require a strong bite and lots of chewing. Swallowing difficulties may affect the choices of some elderly people.
- Reduced taste and smell acuity in the elderly (see Chapter 3) tends to increase the consumption of sugary and salty foods.
- Therapeutic diets; the personal availability of some foods may be increased or decreased in some older people because of an increased likelihood of following a therapeutic diet to treat a chronic disease, e.g. chronic renal failure or the maturity onset form of diabetes mellitus.
- Increased avoidances of a range of foods occurs because a perceived increase in the likelihood of suffering from digestive problems (e.g. flatulence, diarrhoea or indigestion) in response to some spicy, acidic or fibre-rich foods.
- Lack of appetite due to effects of drugs, illness or depression may reduce the availability of all foods. Psychological problems may increase the 'availability' of alcohol.

Aids to food selection

Food groups have long been used as tools in nutrition education in order to help consumers ensure that they select a diet that contains adequate amounts of essential nutrients.

The four food group plan

The four food group plan is the most familiar and widely used. Foods are broken down into four broad categories, each supplying some of the components of an adequate diet:

- the meat group
- the milk group
- the fruit and vegetable group
- the cereals group.

Consumers can ensure an adequate supply of all the essential nutrients by ensuring that they eat set minimum daily portions from each of these four groups. For most of the population in industrialised countries, dietary adequacy is now almost taken for granted; those who consume sufficient calories and eat a range of foods generally meet their minimum needs for essential nutrients without the necessity to take conscious measures to ensure adequacy. Nutritional change that may delay or reduce the risk of chronic degenerative diseases is now the priority in nutrition education for adults and older children. Adequacy is not necessarily quite so assured in older people. A large minority of very elderly people are underweight; inactivity and low basal metabolic rate may reduce energy needs very considerably so that the amount of food eaten may be insufficient to meet all other nutrient needs unless the nutrient density of the diet is high. Amongst some groups of elderly people, undernutrition may be all too prevalent (see Chapter 5). Such factors mean that adequacy assumes a greater priority in nutrition education for the elderly than it currently does for younger adults.

The Food Guide Pyramid

The Food Guide Pyramid, shown in Figure 2.4, has now superseded food groups in nutrition education in the USA and reflects the changing emphasis in nutrition education. When used as a guide to food selection, the pyramid should not only ensure dietary adequacy but also promote a dietary pattern that is expected to reduce or delay the degenerative, diet-related diseases. The major limitation of food groups was that they did not indicate the relative amounts of foods from the different groups; they merely indicated minimum portions consistent with the assurance of adequacy. The pyramid is a recognisable development of the four food group plan but also gives a clear visual message about the quantitative contribution from the food groups. A British version of the Food Guide Pyramid has been produced. It is essentially the same as that shown in Figure 2.4 with just a couple of minor differences, namely:

A Guide to Daily Food Choices

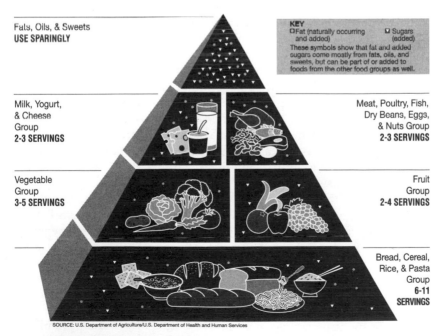

Fats, Oils, & Sweets
USE SPARINGLY

KEY
☐ Fat (naturally occurring and added)   ▨ Sugars (added)
These symbols show that fat and added sugars come mostly from fats, oils, and sweets, but can be part of or added to foods from the other food groups as well.

Milk, Yogurt, & Cheese Group
2-3 SERVINGS

Meat, Poultry, Fish, Dry Beans, Eggs, & Nuts Group
2-3 SERVINGS

Vegetable Group
3-5 SERVINGS

Fruit Group
2-4 SERVINGS

Bread, Cereal, Rice, & Pasta Group
6-11 SERVINGS

SOURCE: U.S. Department of Agriculture/U.S. Department of Health and Human Services

Figure 2.4 The Food Guide Pyramid – a guide to daily food choices.
Source: U.S. Department of Agriculture

- the fruits and vegetables are shown as a single group on the second tier with a combined 5–9 servings
- potatoes are included with the bread and cereals rather than with the fruits and vegetables.

At the base of the Food Guide Pyramid are the cereals, indicating that starchy cereals and potatoes should be the staple components of the diet and provide the bulk of the calories. Cereals should be accompanied by large amounts of fruits and vegetables, which are often relatively low in energy but high in other nutrients. Animal foods (and vegetarian substitutes) like milk products, eggs, meat, fish, nuts and pulses are seen as vital contributors to the nutritional quality and palatability of the diet but should be used relatively sparingly because they are often high in fat, saturated fat, cholesterol and calories. At the top of the pyramid are the fats, sweets, soft drinks and alcoholic drinks. They are important contributors to the palatability of the diet, but provide few nutrients, only calories in the form of sugar, fat and alcohol. They should be used frugally, in the minimum amounts necessary to produce a varied, interesting and palatable diet. The likely sources of fats and added sugars within the various food groups are also indicated by circular and triangular symbols respectively. Both symbols are densely scattered in the fats, oils and sweets compartment. The fat symbol is quite densely scattered throughout the animal products tier, reflecting the fact that many of these foods naturally contain high levels of fat; it is more sparsely distributed in the vegetable and cereal group indicating that fat may be added to these foods during their preparation. The symbol for added sugars is lightly distributed throughout the milk, fruit and cereal groups to reflect the fact that sugar may be added to certain foods within these categories.

In addition to providing a visual image of the 'ideal' dietary pattern, the pyramid is supplemented with more precise guidance on the numbers of specified portions from within each category that should comprise diets of various calorific contents. The approximate numbers of portions from the various categories that should comprise a diet to provide the Estimated Average Requirement (EAR) for elderly adults in the UK is shown in Table 2.6.

The pyramid would seem to be most useful in nutrition education in schools and colleges. When used as a visual qualitative guide to aid in food selection it may be useful in influencing the dietary habits of the whole population. Most nutritionists would accept the broad dietary pattern suggested by the pyramid even though many may have some reservations about the more detailed quantitative suggestions. The pyramid may be particularly useful in counteracting some current misapprehensions, for example the negative image of starchy foods and the belief that the ideal diet contains large amounts of 'high protein' animal foods. Some of these misapprehensions are partly the result of earlier nutrition education and may thus be particularly prevalent amongst older people. We do however question the wisdom of trying to persuade older people to abandon the practices of a lifetime and rigorously apply the prescriptive quantitative guidelines of the pyramid in their food selection.

Table 2.6 Using the Food Guide Pyramid to provide the estimated energy requirements of elderly UK adults

	Men	Women
EAR (kcal)	2100–2330	1810–1900
EAR (MJ)	8.77–9.71	7.61–7.96
Bread group	9	7
Vegetable group	4	3–4
Fruit group	3	2–3
Milk group	2–3	2–3
Meat group	2	2

These figures are intended only to be an approximate guide: the exact calorie content would be very dependent upon extent to which fats, sweets and oils are consumed and factors like the fat content of any milk used, the leanness of meat, whether white fish or oily fish is used and whether vegetables are boiled or fried.

Portions (as in USDA, 1992)

1 slice bread, ½ cup cooked rice, pasta or cereal, 25 g ready-to-eat cereal.

½ cup chopped raw or cooked vegetables, 1 cup leafy raw vegetables.

1 piece fruit, ½ cup canned fruit, ¼ cup dried fruit, ¾ cup fruit juice.

1 cup milk or yoghurt, 40–50 g cheese.

70–80 g cooked lean meat, poultry or fish; an egg or ½ a cup of cooked beans counts as about ⅓ of a serving.

The Food Guide Plate

In the UK, the Health Education Authority (HEA, 1994) has published a new *National Food Guide*. This guide (see Figure 2.5) uses as its visual image a plate divided between five food groups:

- about 30% of the plate is allocated to the fruit and vegetable group
- about 30% of the plate to the bread, potato and cereal group
- around 15% of the area is allocated to the milk and dairy group
- 15% is allocated to the meat, fish and pulses
- the remaining 10% is allocated to fatty and sugary foods.

The general dietary structure suggested by the Food Guide Plate is very similar to that suggested by the Food Guide Pyramid. In this guide however, specific recommendations about portion numbers are avoided because it is felt that this is potentially misleading and confusing, given the large variability in individual energy requirements.

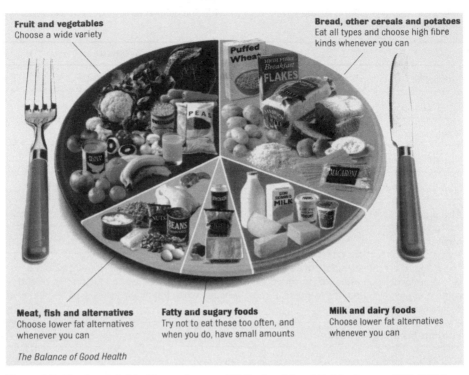

Fruit and vegetables
Choose a wide variety

Bread, other cereals and potatoes
Eat all types and choose high fibre kinds whenever you can

Meat, fish and alternatives
Choose lower fat alternatives whenever you can

Fatty and sugary foods
Try not to eat these too often, and when you do, have small amounts

Milk and dairy foods
Choose lower fat alternatives whenever you can

The Balance of Good Health

Figure 2.5 The Food Guide Plate – the new UK National Food Guide. Source: HEA (1994)

Effecting dietary change

The communication process

When a nutrition education or other health promotion programme is being designed the four components of the communication process listed below need to be considered.

THE SOURCE OF THE ADVICE

Is this source likely to be regarded as credible and reliable by the target group? Some examples of factors that might affect the credibility of the source are:

- how official or expert the source is considered to be
- the perceived impartiality of the source – health claims by a manufacturer for its own product might be viewed with suspicion
- the perceived credibility of the source's experience of the circumstances of the target group – being very young might impair the credibility of the source for older people.

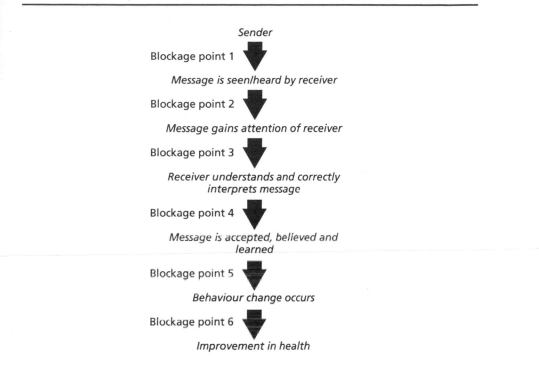

Sender

Blockage point 1

Message is seen/heard by receiver

Blockage point 2

Message gains attention of receiver

Blockage point 3

Receiver understands and correctly interprets message

Blockage point 4

Message is accepted, believed and learned

Blockage point 5

Behaviour change occurs

Blockage point 6

Improvement in health

Figure 2.6 Steps in the process by which a nutrition education message leads to beneficial change in behaviour and potential blockage points

THE MESSAGE ITSELF

Is the message clear, correct, believable and realistic? Has it been framed in a way that will attract the target groups, attention and be understood and believed by them?

THE CHANNEL OR VEHICLE FOR TRANSMITTING THE MESSAGE

Has an appropriate channel been selected, e.g. radio, television, newspaper or poster advertisements, leaflets provided at a doctor's surgery or community centre, speakers addressing groups or one-to-one counselling? What channel is most likely to reach the target group and which vehicle is most likely to influence their behaviour? What is the most cost-effective vehicle for transmitting the message to the target group?

THE RECEIVER OR TARGET FOR THE MESSAGE

What are the standards of education and literacy of the target group, what is their first language? If illiteracy is common then a written message is point-less and English language literature may be less effective than native language literature for some ethnic groups. What are the media habits of the target group? This should help to identify the most useful media channels for transmitting the message. What are the leisure activities and interests of the group, where do they go regularly? A poster aimed at the elderly might have limited impact in a sports centre but more impact in a community centre where an elderly people's lunch or social club meets.

Figure 2.6 summarises some of the stages in the process of a nutrition education or health promotion message leading to changes in behaviour that benefit health. There are potential barriers or blockages to successful nutrition education/health promotion at each of these stages and examples for each of the blockage points are listed below.

Blockage point 1. An inappropriate channel may be chosen and the message will not reach the intended elderly population. Advertisements aimed at elderly people should be scheduled during television or radio programmes that attract older audiences and should be published in newspapers/magazines likely to be read by elderly people. Some simple market research may need to be done to ensure that the message will reach the receiver.

Blockage point 2. The message may not gain the attention of the target group. For example, a poster may not be striking enough or the visual images may not attract elderly people – images of teenage pop idols may not attract the interest of elderly people. Similarly, media programmes/advertisements may be seen as uninteresting by the target group. Programmes, posters, oral presentations and leaflets must be attractive and interesting; they must be appropriate for the elderly.

Blockage point 3. The message may not be understood perhaps because the terminology is inappropriate or the message itself unclear. This may result in a blockage at this stage or if the message is misinterpreted it may result in an inappropriate behaviour change. For example, a message to increase dietary fibre may result in an inappropriate behaviour change if the nature and sources of dietary fibre are misunderstood. Ideally, any promotional material should be piloted with a representative group of elderly people to identify potential problems with terminology, understanding or interpretation.

Blockage point 4. The message may not be believed or, if it is too complex and not reinforced, it may be forgotten. The source may not be perceived as reliable – perhaps the speaker was too young and inexperienced to be credible to an elderly audience. The message may be inconsistent with existing beliefs – advice to increase starchy foods may be inconsistent with the belief that they are fattening or advice to reduce consumption of meat and cheese may be inconsistent with their images as sources of 'vital first class protein'.

Blockage point 5. The required change of behaviour may be difficult or impossible for the receiver to implement. For example, the change may be beyond the economic means of many elderly people or lack of 'gatekeeper availability' may make it difficult for the receiver to change (see earlier in the chapter).

Blockage point 6. The message may be wrong, inappropriately targeted or misunderstood (see blockage point 3). Most of the nutrition education guidelines that have been widely promoted in recent years have been written primarily for the benefit of young and middle-aged adults and may not be particularly appropriate for older people. For example, in the large minority of very elderly people who are underweight or have poor appetite the nutritional priority is to ensure an adequate intake of energy and essential

Table 2.7 Some criteria for judging whether a nutrition education or other health promotion intervention for older adults is justified by available evidence (after Webb, 1992 and 1995)

1 Have clear dietary objectives been set; are they realistic for older people and have all foreseeable aspects of their likely impact been considered?
2 Is there strong evidence that a large proportion of elderly people will gain significant benefits from the proposed change or is evidence of likely benefit confined to studies using younger people?
3 Has there been active and adequate consideration of whether the intended change, or any consequential change, might have adverse effects upon a significant number of elderly people?
4 Have the evaluations of risk and benefit been made holistically? Reductions in risk markers or even in a particular disease are not ends in themselves. Likewise, evaluation of risk should not be confined to possible direct physiological harm but should also include for example, economic, psychological or social repercussions.
5 Has the possibility of targeting intervention to likely gainers been fully explored so as to maximise the benefit to risk ratio? Are elderly people an appropriate target group?
6 Has there been active consideration of how the desired change can be implemented with the minimum disruption to the chosen lifestyle and dietary practices of elderly people.

nutrients – they should be encouraged to eat anything that will help to ensure adequacy; the nutrition education guidelines for chronic disease prevention become largely superfluous.

One of the aims of this book is to review critically the appropriateness of various nutrition education guidelines to the nutritional needs and priorities of older people. Earlier in the chapter it was argued that dietary changes that are ineffective cannot be assumed inevitably to be innocuous; in fact, it is argued that ineffective changes should be regarded as almost inevitably harmful if a truly holistic view is taken. It is therefore not acceptable to assume merely that changes designed to benefit younger people should be automatically applied to older people in the belief that though they do no good neither will they do any harm. Webb (1992, 1995) has suggested some criteria that might be applied to judge whether any particular 'intervention' is justified by available evidence; these are summarised in Table 2.7.

Factors that influence the likelihood of dietary change

Fieldhouse (1986) lists a series of factors that will affect the likelihood of any dietary change being implemented:

- **The advantage of change and the observability of that advantage.** If a relatively minor dietary change results in immediate, apparent benefits then this increases the likelihood of permanent adoption; if the benefits of change are not immediately apparent or speculative or if the change itself is seen as having a major negative impact (e.g. restricting favoured foods, increased cost or increased preparation time) then this will decrease the likelihood of implementation.

- **Its compatibility with existing beliefs, cultural values and culinary style.** Advice that is compatible with existing beliefs and behaviour is more likely to be implemented than that which is contrary to these beliefs and behaviours (e.g. advising a pious person to break the dietary rules of their religion has a low probability of success).
- **Its complexity.** The more difficult it is to understand or to implement any change the lower is the probability of it being implemented.
- **Its trialability.** If advice is easy to try out on a 'one off' basis, people are more likely to try it out than if it requires more commitment such as the learning of a new preparation method or buying new catering equipment. Trying something out is the first step on the way to permanently adopting the advice.

Webb (1995) uses the example of a change that will result in the cure of a deficiency disease as one that has a high probability of being made. The major advantages of such a change are usually readily apparent within a short period of time and can often be observed in others who have already made the change. The disadvantages of such a change may be small (e.g. incorporation of a nutrient-rich or fortified food in the diet or even the consumption of a nutrient supplement). Such a change is also easy to understand and implement. It can usually be tried without any long-term commitment and the rapid and obvious benefits act as a strong positive reinforcement to continue with the change in diet.

Likewise, where adoption or partial adoption of a therapeutic diet gives rapid symptomatic relief this will also act as powerful, positive reinforcement, encouraging clients to continue with adopted measures and perhaps adopt more of the recommended measures. For example, if adoption of a low protein diet gives symptomatic relief from uraemia (headache, drowsiness, nausea, anorexia and vomiting) in patients with chronic renal failure this will encourage patients to persevere with the diet despite its relative complexity and restrictiveness. Such a diet may also slow the rate of deterioration in renal function and if explained to the patient this could act as an extra incentive to adopt the dietary advice. This slowing in the progress of renal failure is still controversial and will certainly not be so readily apparent to the patient, so by itself would not be as powerful an incentive as any symptomatic relief. Similarly, if increased water and fibre intakes in the elderly relieve constipation, symptoms of dehydration or give symptomatic relief from minor bowel disorders (e.g. diverticulosis or haemorrhoids) these benefits will act as a positive reinforcement; putative long-term benefits such as reducing the risk of bowel cancer or heart disease may be less persuasive.

Where dietary advice to older people is directed towards restoration of nutritional adequacy or the treatment of an established disease then, if thoughtfully constructed this should have a relatively high likelihood of adoption especially if there are immediate and apparent symptomatic benefits.

Where dietary advice is geared towards reducing symptomless risk markers (e.g. serum cholesterol) and reducing the later risk of chronic disease in currently healthy subjects then the balance of advantage may be very different and it may prove more difficult to persuade people to implement changes (see Chapter 4 for a discussion of strategies for risk reduction). The benefits of change are not immediately apparent: they are often predicted to accrue some time after introduction of the change; they are often perceived as speculative with some expert opinion arguing against even the long-term benefits of change. Anecdotal observations may also tend to confound the predictions of the experts. There will be examples of 'healthy eaters' who nevertheless develop diet-related diseases and those who ignore dietary guidelines but remain healthy well into old age. This anecdotal tendency may be compounded by the tendency of people to adopt practices they perceive as healthy when they start to become concerned about their health. In such a case adoption of a healthy diet may apparently immediately precede the onset of overt symptoms and so may even appear causative.

Conversely, the changes required to meet current nutrition education guidelines may be perceived as having immediate and major disadvantages such as the restriction of highly palatable sugary, salty and fatty foods and their partial replacement with bland, starchy and fibrous foods. Increasing fear and guilt about 'inappropriate' eating behaviours may be one way of altering the balance of advantage of implementing change. Thus a first heart attack can persuade people to adopt strict cholesterol-lowering diets and the onset of serious lung disease may persuade people to give up smoking. However, health promotion that tries to harness such fear of death and disease as a means of inducing dietary/lifestyle change in healthy people serves to focus people's attention upon death and disease. It may have some negative impact upon quality of life. If such 'health promotion' succeeds in generating fear and guilt without changing behaviour, or results in changes that ultimately prove not to be beneficial, then its impact will be totally negative. Similarly, increased feedback by regular monitoring of risk markers may improve compliance but it may also increase the client's preoccupation with death and disease.

Some other specific points that may particularly reduce the likelihood of dietary change being implemented by older people are listed below.

- The food beliefs of older people may be more traditional and less flexible than those of younger people.
- If older people live alone, or just with their spouses, or have limited mobility, any change that requires more preparation or shopping effort, or requires the acquisition of new skills or utensils is likely to be perceived as particularly disadvantageous.
- Many elderly people are relatively poor and so any change that requires extra expenditure upon food may be seen as particularly disadvantageous.
- People are said to adapt gradually to foods prepared with less salt and perhaps sugar; this process of adaptation may be impaired by declining taste acuity in older people. Likewise, increases in dietary fibre may initially produce adverse gastrointestinal symptoms (e.g. flatulence, diarrhoea) and

older people may be particularly sensitive to these effects. Older people may need a longer trial period to adapt or may simply not adapt to these changes as well as younger people. In general ageing leads to a loss of adaptability.

Beliefs, attitudes and enabling factors

The factors that influence whether a received health promotion/nutrition education recommendation is actually implemented can be broken down into two major categories – beliefs and enabling factors. An individual's beliefs about diet and/or health will clearly influence their judgement about whether a suggested change is beneficial. If one is seeking to persuade people to modify their behaviour in order to reduce the risk of a particular disease, then first they must believe that they are susceptible to the disease, secondly that the consequences are serious and finally that it can be prevented (Becker, 1984). If we take heart disease as an example then in order to make a judgement to modify their behaviour and so avoid heart disease, the subjects must believe:

- that they are at risk from heart disease (susceptible)
- that heart disease can kill or disable (the consequences are serious)
- that if they stop smoking/lose excess weight/take more exercise/change their diet, the risk is reduced (prevention is possible).

It is not only the beliefs of the subjects themselves that will influence their judgements but also the influences of family, friends, colleagues, teachers, religious leaders, health workers and others. Ajzen and Fishbein (1980) described these influences from the beliefs and attitudes of others as the perceived social pressure or the 'subjective norm'. Health education campaigns that are directed solely at elderly people may fail if they do not change the subjective norm and so leave the beliefs and advice from those who influence elderly people unaltered and contrary to that of the nutrition education/health promotion message. This will be a particular problem where the nutrition education advice for the bulk of the adult population differs from that offered to elderly people. If the whole population is bombarded with warnings about the dangers of being overweight and advice about ways of losing weight then 'overweight is bad, low body weight/losing weight is good' becomes the subjective norm. In very elderly people, avoiding underweight and maintaining nutritional adequacy may be the nutritional priority but it may be difficult for those giving dietary advice to modify their beliefs when dealing with elderly clients or even for elderly people to accept that the subjective norm may not always be entirely appropriate for them.

Individual beliefs and the subjective norm will affect a person's judgement of any particular recommendation and thus affect their behaviour intentions. A host of 'enabling factors' will influence whether or not any intention or wish to change behaviour is translated into actual behaviour change. These enabling factors may come under a variety of headings such as:

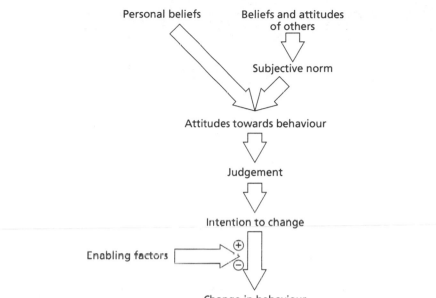

Figure 2.7 A scheme to illustrate how beliefs, attitudes and enabling factors interact to determine whether a recommended change results in actual behaviour change (after Hubley, 1993)

- Physical resources – is the change physically possible for the person (e.g. can they obtain the recommended foods or have they the implements/facilities necessary for their preparation)?
- Financial resources – can they afford to make the recommended change?
- Personal resources – have they the skills and mobility necessary to implement the recommended change?

Many of these enabling factors were discussed earlier in the chapter under the 'hierarchy of availabilities' (Figure 2.1). In this model of food selection it is assumed that a host of factors, at several levels, limit any individual's practical freedom of dietary choice and thus their ability to implement any recommended change.

Figure 2.7 shows a diagrammatic representation of how beliefs, the subjective norm, attitudes and enabling factors interact to determine whether any recommended dietary change is actually implemented. The one element of this model that has not been addressed so far is 'attitude' to change. People may be convinced that a health/nutrition education message is applicable to them, the subjective norm may favour change and the enabling factors may permit them to make the recommended change. However, change may still not occur; they may make a conscious decision to accept the risks associated with current behaviour, perhaps because of the perceived adverse effect of change on their quality of life. In some cases the quality of life being experienced may be so low that the prospect of an extension of life is actually a disincentive to change.

Some physiological consequences of ageing and their relationship to nutrition

Overview and aims of the chapter

There is measurable age-related deterioration in the functioning of most systems of the body (see Figure 3.1). The rate of deterioration varies greatly between different systems. According to Green (1994), these changes are usually earliest and fastest in those systems where there is no replacement of dead cells (e.g. brain, muscle and heart) but slower and later in those where continual replacement occurs (e.g. red cells and intestinal epithelium). Generally, more complex functions involving co-ordination are more affected than simple ones: note for example, that in Figure 3.1, the decline in reaction time is rapid compared with the fall in nerve conduction velocity.

The rate of age-related deterioration also varies greatly between different individuals. The heterogeneous nature of the elderly population is something that is stressed several times in this book; a group of elderly people of the same chronological age will vary substantially in their ages as determined by physiological and psychological criteria. Some deterioration in physiological functioning with age is inevitable, but the rate will be affected by lifestyle and

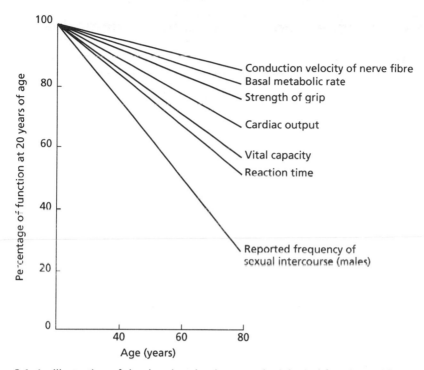

Figure 3.1 An illustration of the deterioration in some physiological functions with age. Source: Green (1994)

environmental influences (including diet). Part of the individual variation in the effects of ageing is due to innate genetic differences but some (in some cases perhaps most) is due to differences in these environmental and lifestyle influences. It is therefore, potentially alterable by changes in diet, lifestyle and environment. For example ageing professional athletes, no matter how hard they train, inevitably reach an age when they can no longer compete with the best of the younger athletes. Nevertheless, these ageing professional athletes can greatly outperform almost all of their peers and can still outperform all but the most highly trained and talented amongst a much younger population.

In this chapter, some of the age-related anatomical, physiological and biochemical changes in the various systems of the body are briefly overviewed and their functional consequences discussed. More detailed accounts of the physiology of ageing may be found in Kenney (1989) and Green (1994). Where appropriate, the likely role of dietary and lifestyle factors in accelerating or retarding these changes is also outlined. Topics that are considered of particular relevance to a text on nutrition and the elderly have been selected for more extended discussion, namely:

- the effects of ageing upon physical fitness and strength
- fluid balance and renal function in the elderly
- ageing and immune function
- ageing of the skeleton and osteoporosis.

Effects of ageing on body systems – summaries

The muscular system

As people get older, their total muscle mass declines due to both a reduction in the number of muscle fibres and a reduction in the size of muscle fibres. There is a pronounced tendency for muscles to become infiltrated with fat and cross sectional views of muscles in elderly people show that much of the lean muscle tissue has been replaced by fat. There is also a decline in the number of motorneurones supplying muscles.

This decline in muscle mass and number of muscle fibres results in a decline in strength with age. The rate of loss of muscle fibres is greater than that of motorneurones and so the size of motor units is decreased in the elderly. This means that more motor units have to be employed in order to perform a given task and this is perceived as an increase in effort required by the subject. The decline in lean muscle mass is probably the reason for the decline in basal metabolic rate in older people, which reduces their energy requirements and which, if not matched by increased nutrient density, predisposes them to nutrient deficiencies (see Chapter 5).

As discussed later, much of this age-related decline in muscle mass and strength represents a form of disuse atrophy. It can be minimised and to some extent reversed, even in very elderly people, by appropriate exercise programmes.

The skeleton

There is an increase in the rate of bone resorption in middle-aged and elderly people and this leads to a decline in bone mass and bone strength with age. The rate of bone loss accelerates in women around the time of the menopause. Osteoporosis, the tendency of bones to fracture when subjected to relatively minor trauma, is much more common in elderly women than it is in elderly men. There is calcification of the joints and a loss of elasticity of cartilage with age which leads to increased stiffening of the joints and a loss of flexibility. Thinning of cartilage in the weight-bearing areas leads to increased likelihood of the elderly experiencing osteoarthritic pain.

Inactivity almost certainly plays a part in increasing the rate of bone loss and thus in increasing the propensity to osteoporotic fracture. Inactivity also plays a part in reducing the flexibility of joints. The role of other dietary factors and particularly dietary calcium in the aetiology of osteoporosis is more controversial and is discussed later in the chapter.

The skin

There is a loss of elasticity of the fibrous elements of skin and dehydration of the ground substance that leads to wrinkling of the skin of older people. There is a loss of hair. Reduced activity and density of melanocytes (pigment producing cells) leads to greying of the hair and pallor of the skin. Loss of subcutaneous adipose tissue may reduce the effectiveness of thermal insulation and may be a factor in the propensity of older people to hypothermia. There is reduced function of the sweat and sebaceous glands. Wounds heal more slowly in the elderly.

Some of the age-related changes in skin are attributable to the chronic and cumulative effects of exposure to the harmful radiation in sunlight. Slower wound healing is of considerable clinical significance – it increases the risk of wounds becoming infected and may extend the hospital stay of elderly, injury and surgery patients; malnutrition also delays wound healing.

The pulmonary system

There is a decrease in the elasticity of the lungs and the chest wall becomes less compliant with age – this increases the work that is required to breathe. There is a reduction in the size of the alveoli, reducing the surface area available for gas exchange. There is an increase in the residual volume of the lungs (the air that remains in the lungs after full expiration) and a decrease in the vital capacity (the amount of gas that can be expired after a maximal inspiration).

These changes do not normally impair the ability to supply oxygen to the tissues at rest but they do limit the capacity of the system during heavy exercise. A large decline in muscle strength may also affect the respiratory muscles and thus the ability to cough and expectorate. This may predispose elderly people to pneumonia and these effects may compound with effects upon the immune system. Malnutrition has similar effects upon both strength and immune function. Lung diseases, including pneumonia, become an increasingly prominent cause of death in the elderly.

The cardiovascular system

There is a tendency for heart muscle to be replaced by fibrous connective tissue leading to reduced elasticity of the ageing heart. There may also be fibrosis of the heart valves. The ventricular volume at the end of diastole (cardiac relaxation) is increased, suggesting greater filling of the ventricles with blood. There is decreased compliance (elasticity) of arteries and partial occlusion by atherosclerosis.

The resting stroke volume, cardiac output and heart rate may all be unaltered in the ageing heart – although note that the degree of stretch (the end diastolic volume) required to achieve the stroke volume is increased. The maximum heart rate, stroke volume and heart rate all decline with age. The maximum heart rate at any given age can be roughly predicted by the equation:

Maximum heart rate (beats/min) = 220 – age (in years)

The systolic blood pressure tends to rise because of decreased compliance (elasticity) of the aorta and diastolic blood pressure tends to increase due to increases in the total peripheral resistance to blood flow.

The renal system

There is a decrease in the weight of the kidney with age and a loss of functional units (nephrons). There is a decrease in renal perfusion and glomerular filtration rate and thus an impaired ability to eliminate nitrogenous waste products (urea). There is an increase in the renal threshold for glucose, i.e. glucose starts to appear in the urine at higher blood concentrations in older people. Considerable loss of renal function can occur before it becomes symptomatic under normal conditions, although the ability to produce very concentrated or very dilute urine is reduced (see later in the chapter). If glomerular filtration falls far enough, then blood urea and creatinine levels rise giving symptoms of chronic renal failure.

The alimentary system

MOUTH

There is a decrease in the number of taste buds with age which leads to reduce taste acuity and perhaps to increased use of salt and sugar. There is a reduction in the secretion of saliva which may compound with other factors to cause difficulties with swallowing (see Chapter 8 for discussion of swallowing difficulties). In affluent countries, ageing is associated with lack of teeth, which clearly impairs biting and chewing abilities. These biting and chewing problems are partially compensated for by dental prostheses; the effectiveness of this compensation will depend very much upon how well these dentures fit and the general state of oral health.

In 1988, more than half of the over 65s in the UK had no natural teeth and this figure increased to well over 75% in the over 75s. These figures represent substantial improvements on the situation in 1968. In 1968 in the 65–74 year age group about three quarters of people had no natural teeth but by 1988 this had dropped to just under half (DH, 1992a). It is projected that these improvements in the dental health of the elderly will continue, so that by the end of the century, only around a quarter of elderly people will be without any natural teeth. These changes point to the need for changes in the dental service provision for elderly people. Poor dental health can have a marked effect upon the food choices and nutritional status of elderly people. Given the past experience of most elderly people having no natural teeth, dental monitoring, dental education and provision of dental care for the elderly may be neglected.

STOMACH

There is atrophy of both the mucosal and muscle layers of the stomach with age. There is reduced gastric acid secretion which may predispose to gastrointestinal infection and may reduce the efficiency of iron absorption.

Pernicious anaemia is more common in the elderly; this is due to autoimmune destruction of the cells in the stomach producing the intrinsic factor necessary for vitamin B_{12} absorption.

SMALL INTESTINE

The intestinal villi become shorter and broader and this reduces the area of the absorptive surface. The efficiency of absorption of several nutrients may decrease with age, although the effect upon dietary nutrient requirements is generally not well established.

LARGE INTESTINE

There is atrophy of the mucosal and muscle layers and a weakening of the colon wall. Ageing is associated with a decrease in peristaltic movement throughout the alimentary tract but particularly in the colon and rectum. Changes in the large intestine compound with other factors to increase the prevalence of constipation in the elderly. The weakening of the muscle layers may lead to diverticular disease; a ballooning out of the intestinal wall to form a pouch or diverticulum, that may become inflamed. Increased intakes of dietary fibre (non-starch polysaccharide), together with prevention of dehydration and reasonable levels of physical activity, are seen as important factors in the prevention and alleviation of constipation (see Chapter 8). Dietary fibre also gives symptomatic relief in diverticular disease.

THE LIVER

There is a decrease in the size and cellularity of the liver with age. This may lead to a considerable reduction in the capacity for drug metabolism or indeed for the metabolism of other ingested toxicants (see Chapter 5).

The immune system

There is a general shrinkage of lymphoid tissue in the elderly (the spleen, thymus and lymph nodes). There is reduced T-cell function and to a lesser extent B–cell function. This leads to increased susceptibility to infection, autoimmune disease and cancer. In general, the cell-mediated immunity is more affected than humoural (antibody) immunity. Malnutrition gives rise to deleterious effects on the immune system that are similar to the changes associated with ageing (see later in this chapter).

The endocrine system

The secretion of many hormones appears to be relatively unaffected by age. Secretion of the pituitary gonadotrophins increases in the elderly due to a diminution in negative feedback because of the declining output of sex hormones from the gonads. In women, this decline in sex hormone output is more pronounced and occurs relatively sharply at the menopause. Hormone replacement therapy (HRT) seeks to replace the missing oestrogenic hormones in postmenopausal women in order to reduce the symptoms of the menopause and the postmenopausal deterioration in some body systems particularly the postmenopausal acceleration in bone loss. Decreased tissue sensitivity to some hormones occurs with age, e.g. insulin (see relevant sections in Chapters 4 and 8). There is reduced efficiency of conversion of vitamin D to the active hormone 1,25 dihydroxycholecalciferol in the kidney; this, together with reduced exposure of the skin to sunlight, may make some elderly people prone to symptoms of vitamin D deficiency, osteomalacia.

Sense organs

VISION

There is a loss of elasticity of the lens of the eye, leading to a reduced ability to accommodate when viewing close objects (e.g. when reading). The near point gets further away with age; people become far-sighted as they get older. The opacity of the lens increases with age, increasing the likelihood of cataracts. There is a loss of photoreceptive cells in the retina. There is overgrowth of blood vessels in the retina; these may leak and cause degeneration of the retina (retinopathy). There is a general loss of visual acuity with age. There is fatty infiltration of the area around the cornea which presents as a white border around the cornea – the arcus senilis. Both cataract and retinopathy are accelerated in diabetes and glucose intolerance and this seems to be the result of prolonged hyperglycaemia (see Chapter 8).

About 97% of Britons over the age of 65 years wear glasses. Many elderly people still have difficulty with their eyesight even when wearing corrective lenses – around 15% of 65–69-year-olds, rising to over 40% of the over 85s (DH, 1992a).

HEARING

There is a general deterioration in the auditory system with age, leading to the following functional changes:

* increased auditory threshold particularly at higher frequencies
* narrowing of the range of audible frequencies, with a substantial loss of higher frequencies
* loss of ability to locate sounds accurately.

Accumulation of wax can be a cause of hearing loss in the elderly.

Around 10% of Britons aged over 65 years wear a hearing aid and many more elderly people have hearing difficulties but do not use a hearing aid. Probably a quarter of those aged 65–69 years have hearing difficulties, rising progressively to around 60% of the over 85s (DH, 1992a).

OTHER SENSES

There is a reduction in the sense of smell with age and this together with loss of taste acuity may reduce the pleasure gained from food and may also increase the chances of stale or spoiled food being consumed. Cutaneous senses are diminished with age, there are increases in the pain and temperature thresholds and reduced ability to discriminate by touch. The accuracy and sensitivity of proprioceptor mechanisms diminishes with age (proprioceptors are those sensory receptors that provide information about body position and movement). This latter effect may contribute to the risk of falling, the major cause of accidental death in the elderly.

The brain

There is a slow loss of brain weight with age that amounts to about 7% of the total brain weight between 20–80 years. Neurones are lost throughout life but the rate of loss is highest in the developing brain; although the absolute number of neurones losses sound very large, they amount to only a few per cent of the original total over the whole lifetime. There is a reduction in the area of the cerebral cortex that is brought about by a flattening of the surface ridges (gyri) and a broadening of the furrows (sulci). In the neurones, there is a degeneration or 'dying back' of axons and a loss of neuronal microtubules. There is increased appearance of densely arranged helices of microtubules, neurofibrillary tangles, which are prominent in patients with Alzheimer's disease. There are increasing numbers of areas of localised degeneration, particularly in the cerebral cortex – the senile plaques.

There is a decline in the cerebral blood flow with age and, in the very elderly, blood flow may be close to the minimum level necessary for full neuronal function.

Some of the functional changes in the nervous system are listed below.

- There is a delay, or in some cases absence of reflexes in the elderly. Reaction times are increased in the elderly.
- The sleep patterns of elderly people differ from those of younger people. The elderly are 'lighter sleepers'. The elderly may take longer to fall asleep, they tend to wake more frequently during the night and to stay awake for longer at each awakening.
- There are changes in cognitive functions in the elderly and Kenney (1989) attributes these changes to two factors:
    a loss of neurones and synapses
    a reduction in the speed of neuronal processes.

In simple attention tests then, older people often perform almost as well as the young, although their attention span is shorter. In more complex situations, (e.g. where there are distracting influences or where attention must be divided between two tasks) the elderly perform much less well than young adults. There is a decline, with age, in the performance in short-term memory tests.

There is a reduced speed of learning in older people. There is a marked decline in the speed at which psychomotor tasks can be accomplished in the elderly.

Whole body changes

There is a loss of height with age – approximately 1 cm per decade from 30 years onwards. This may complicate the interpretation of anthropometric data in the elderly (see Chapter 6).

There is a marked change in body composition with age – the proportions of lean tissue and bone decline and the proportion of fat increases.

There is a decline in the basal metabolic rate with age. This is probably a function of the decline in lean body mass and has important nutritional implications (see Chapter 5).

The speed of homeostatic regulation is reduced – it takes longer for an elderly person to restore the equilibrium position after the imposition of any constraint. Some examples are given below.

* In response to cold stress old people tend to start shivering later and in response to heat stress they sweat later. Old people are more susceptible to hypothermia because they have a reduced basal metabolic rate, less ability to generate heat by voluntary activity and shivering and reduced insulation because of the changes in the skin outlined earlier.
* There is an impaired capacity to restore acid-base balance if it is disturbed due to reduced buffering capacity, diminished respiratory responses to acid-base disturbances, and an impaired ability of the kidney to eliminate excess acid or base.
* There is a decline in the efficiency of the mechanisms regulating salt and water balance and these are discussed later in this chapter.

Effects of ageing upon fitness and strength

Aerobic fitness is a measure of the capacity of the lungs and circulatory system to deliver oxygen to the muscles and other tissues during maximal exercise. In untrained subjects and older people it would normally be estimated from the heart rate of subjects whilst undergoing submaximal exercise loads such as cycling on a bicycle ergometer or walking/running on a treadmill. It has traditionally been said that measurable increases in aerobic fitness require training programmes of specified minimum duration, intensity and frequency; as a rough rule of thumb they should raise heart rate to 60–70% of maximum for durations of 20 minutes on three occasions each week. There are, however, several other short term benefits of exercise that will accrue at intensities and durations well below those required to increase aerobic fitness:

* increased muscle strength
* improved endurance of both individual muscle groups and the cardiopulmonary system

- increases in flexibility; the range of movements that can be safely and comfortably accomplished
- improved psychological wellbeing.

These latter benefits are much more significant for older people than increases in aerobic fitness. Regular exercise, even of fairly low intensity and duration may yield substantial real benefits for older people. Resistance training, aimed at improving the strength of particular muscle groups may also be beneficial. Exercise should help to maintain lean tissue mass, increase total energy expenditure (see Chapter 5) and extend the time that older people remain mobile and able to function independently. It is generally assumed that, even in old age, some of the deterioration in function in sedentary people can be reversed by a suitable training programme (Bassey, 1985). There is a substantial body of evidence that in the longer term reduced morbidity and mortality also result from an active lifestyle and this is discussed in Chapter 4.

In the Allied Dunbar National Fitness Survey (1992), it was found that, as one might expect, average aerobic fitness of UK adults of both sexes declined with advancing age. Despite this, there were many elderly people who had aerobic fitness levels higher than some less fit people more than 40 years younger than themselves. For example, the average aerobic fitness of the top 10% of men aged 65–74 years was higher than the average of the bottom 10% of men aged 25–34 years. This survey also found that the loss of muscle strength across the ages was 'dramatic'. Despite this, the authors concluded that much of this loss of strength was not inevitable and was potentially reversible. Almost a fifth of adults in the 65–74 age group, showed significant impairment in the flexibility of their shoulder joints but once again the authors concluded that this limitation could have been prevented or ameliorated. Thus, in this survey, ageing was associated with a substantial decline in aerobic fitness, muscle strength and flexibility but the report's authors suggest that only a relatively minor proportion of this decline is due to age *per se* – 'age is a factor in determining fitness for everyday tasks but not the most important one'. They further concluded that 'much functional disability among older people could be reversed or avoided through continued regular exercise as people grow older'.

Fiatarone *et al.* (1994) specifically addressed the issue of whether some of the age-related deterioration in muscle functioning is indeed potentially reversible. They took 100 frail and very elderly people (mean age 87 years) living in a nursing home and gave them one of the following treatments for a ten-week period:

- a multinutrient diet supplement
- a resistance training programme designed to train and strengthen the hip and knee extensor muscles
- treatments 1 and 2 combined
- placebo treatments (a nutrient-free supplement and some activity that did not involve resistance training).

In this trial, resistance training led to significant increases in muscle strength, walking speed, stair-climbing power and spontaneous physical activity as compared to the unexercised groups. The training also resulted in measurable increases in the cross sectional area of the thigh muscle. It was particularly encouraging that almost all of these frail and very elderly people completed the exercise programme.

Several previous studies had failed to show much improvement in muscle strength with training in frail elderly people (see Fiatarone and Evans, 1993). The resistance training method employed by Fiatarone and her colleagues was of the low repetition, high intensity type that was specifically geared to increasing muscle strength. Aerobic type exercises, employed by some other groups, involve high repetition, low intensity muscle contractions and these are relatively ineffective in increasing muscle strength. Fiatarone and her colleagues used a resistance of 80% of the one repetition maximum (the maximum load that can be lifted once). They increased the resistance throughout the training period as the subject's one repetition maximum increased.

One of the targets in *The health of the nation* is to reduce the death rate from accidents amongst the over 65s by a third over the period 1990–2005 (DH, 1992). Around 4500 over 65s die each year in accidents and although this is a small proportion of total deaths in this age group, they are regarded as 'preventable'. Most accidents in the elderly occur in the home and over two-thirds of these home accidents involve falls and fractures. Muscle weakness is a common feature of elderly 'fallers' and so improvements in muscle strength in the elderly might make a considerable contribution to meeting this target for fatal accident reduction in older people.

In this study by Fiatarone and her colleagues, the nutritional supplements had no significant effect upon their particular outcome measures. Lack of short-term improvement in these measures by nutritional supplements does not of course mean that poor nutritional status does not contribute to the long-term, age-related decline in these measures in some elderly people. Other outcome measures (e.g. immune function) might be expected to be more sensitive to dietary intervention. Nutritional supplements might only be expected to be effective in elderly people whose nutritional status was suboptimal prior to the intervention. Prevalence of suboptimal nutrition might be low amongst relatively healthy elderly people living in a well-managed nursing home.

Bassey (1985) reviewed the evidence then available concerning the benefits of exercise in the elderly. She concluded that although improvements in muscle strength and stamina due to training may be smaller and slower to develop in the elderly than in the young, they still occur. Bassey went on to argue that the benefits of exercise may be of even greater importance in the elderly because they facilitate the everyday activities that are necessary for independent living.

Much of the age-associated decline in performance recorded in the National Fitness Survey represents a form of disuse atrophy caused by the tendency of people to curtail their physical activities as they get older (see Chapter 4). This distinction between the measured deterioration in functioning that is associated with ageing and the deterioration that is an inevitable consequence of ageing should be borne in mind during any discussion of age-related changes (usually deterioration) in physiological functioning. It also needs to be borne in mind when interpreting the age-related changes in risk factors that are discussed in Chapter 4. Note also, that the presence of an age-related disease will accelerate physiological deterioration. Such deterioration is associated with ageing but is not a consequence of ageing *per se* as it does not occur in disease-free older people.

Fluid balance and renal function in the elderly

This topic is reviewed by Kenney (1989). There are considerable anatomical and functional age-related changes in the kidney. As a person ages there is a gradual decline in the weight of the kidney and a decline in the number of functional units (nephrons). There are also substantial reductions in two measurable indices of kidney function, the renal perfusion (renal plasma flow) and the glomerular filtration rate. Thus in an 80-year-old the kidney weight is only about 70% of that in a 40-year-old and the number of functional nephrons has also fallen by about 30%. Both renal plasma flow and glomerular filtration rate decline by about 10% per decade and so typical values in 80-year-olds will be halved as compared to the values typical in young adults.

Most people consume water and salt at levels that are well in excess of their minimum requirements. In elderly people, the minimum requirement for water and the risk of dehydration is increased by a number of factors.

- Water loss through the skin is increased because of thinning of the skin in old age.
- There is reduced ability to produce a concentrated urine. A young adult, under conditions of maximum water conservation, can produce urine that is four times as concentrated as plasma. In the elderly, this capacity falls to less than three times. Elimination of excess solutes (e.g. salt) is thus more expensive in terms of the amount of water needed.
- As people get older there is a decline in the sensitivity of the thirst mechanism. Rolls and Phillips (1990) compared the responses of young and elderly men to dehydration induced by 24 hour water deprivation. At the end of the deprivation period, the increase in plasma concentration was greater in the older men although weight losses were identical in the two groups. However, during a 2 hour rehydration phase, when subjects had drinking water freely available, the average water intake of the elderly men was well under half that of the younger men and subjective estimations of thirst were also much reduced in the older men. Similar findings have been reported when dehydration has been induced by exposure to a hot, dry atmosphere (thermal dehydration). In this latter case, the older men sweated at the same rate as the younger men but showed bigger increases in body temperature and plasma concentration; they also experienced less thirst than the younger men. Rolls and Phillips concluded that the acuity and effectiveness of the thirst drive declines with ageing.
- There may also be physical problems in getting drinks because of poor mobility. Reduced muscle strength makes it difficult for many elderly people, especially elderly women, to rise unaided from a sitting position.

Some elderly people may experience difficulties in drinking (e.g. after a stroke).
- There may be voluntary suppression of fluid intake. Fear of incontinence may cause elderly people to reduce their fluid intake. They may also try to avoid the necessity of getting out of bed during the night, perhaps because of fear of falling.
- Reduced taste sensitivity may lead to increased use of salt in the elderly.

These factors may all contribute to inadequate fluid intake, high fluid losses and increased likelihood of dehydration in the elderly. High prevalence (25%) of mild dehydration has been reported in one group of non-ambulatory geriatric patients but this dehydration was completely eliminated by a routine of regular prompts and assistance with drinks (see Rolls and Phillips, 1990).

At the other extreme, elderly people are also more susceptible to overhydration if given large amounts of fluids and a low sodium diet. Young people have the capacity to produce urine that is ten times more dilute than plasma when they are excreting a high water load. This capacity declines markedly with age and so excretion of a water load is both delayed (because of the reduced glomerular filtration rate) and expensive in terms of salt losses because of this reduced ability to produce very dilute urine.

Dehydration can cause or worsen intestinal problems like constipation, it is a common cause of confusion and may increase susceptibility to hypothermia. Those caring for older people in hospitals or retirement homes should be aware of the increased risk of dehydration. Palatable drinks should be freely available and, particularly in the case of immobile clients, should be directly offered at regular intervals and if necessary they should be given assistance with drinking them. Independent elderly people should be aware of the increased risk of dehydration and encouraged to maintain good fluid intakes (the equivalent of 6–8 glasses of water per day has been suggested).

These changes in fluid balance regulation in the elderly are a good example of the general loss of homeostasis; deviations from the target values become bigger and restoration of the target value takes longer. These changes also need to be borne in mind when fluids are given intravenously to older people or when diuretics are prescribed. Reduced urinary excretion may be but one more factor to consider when calculating drug doses for elderly people.

Chronic Renal Failure (CRF)

Renal function may decline by a very substantial amount before it becomes overtly symptomatic e.g. glomerular filtration rate may fall to around a fifth of its value in a young adult before symptoms become apparent. Nevertheless, in a large number of elderly people, symptomatic chronic renal failure (CRF) does develop. Compared to people aged 20–49 years, the incidence of new cases of CRF is five times higher in the over sixties and ten times higher in the over eighties (Feest *et al.*, 1990).

Renal failure leads to increases in blood levels of urea and creatinine and the high level of blood urea (uraemia) causes nausea, vomiting, headache, drowsiness, pruritus (itching), bone pain, spontaneous bruising, anorexia, etc. As renal function declines further the symptoms worsen, and eventually the patient lapses into an uraemic coma and dies. Once CRF has reached an advanced stage, effective treatment requires long term renal replacement therapy, either some form of dialysis or a kidney transplant. Many elderly patients suitable for renal replacement therapy have been denied these treatments solely because of their age (Feest et al., 1990).

High energy, low protein diets have long been used to give symptomatic relief in CRF. As the kidney fails there is reduced excretion of the urea produced during breakdown of dietary protein (or body protein in wasting subjects). This build-up of urea in blood gives rise to the myriad of unpleasant symptoms listed earlier. The high energy, low protein diet minimises urea production, by minimising protein breakdown and so alleviates the symptoms of uraemia. There is a widespread belief that a low protein diet is not only palliative but that, if started in the early stages of renal failure, actually slows the pathological degeneration of the kidney. It may thus extend the period in which conservative management can be used before either dialysis or transplantation become essential (Lee, 1988; Debenham, 1992). It has even been argued that chronic overconsumption of protein in early adult life may be a contributory factor in the aetiology of CRF (e.g. Rudman, 1988).

The benefit of low protein diets in slowing progress of CRF is still a matter of dispute. Most of the studies suggesting that low protein diets reduce the rate of deterioration of renal function have been relatively small scale, short-term and/or imperfectly controlled. Even if protein restriction does slow the rate of renal deterioration, does the magnitude of this benefit justify the restrictions imposed upon the patients and the likely increase in risk of general malnutrition (Hadfield, 1992)? In the past, dietary restriction was often initiated in asymptomatic patients solely on the basis of biochemical evidence of mild renal insufficiency despite little evidence to justify this early intervention. A critical discussion of these issues may be found in Nahas and Coles (1986).

A recent, large and long-term American cohort study using patients with moderate or more severe renal impairment, did support the belief that moderate protein restriction can slow the progression of CRF in patients with moderate renal insufficiency. More severe restriction of protein intake in those with more advanced renal failure did not appear to offer any additional benefits as compared to moderate restriction (Klahr et al., 1994). These days, diets do tend to be more moderate in their protein restriction than in the past. Previously, some diets aimed at protein intakes that were only a third of the typical allowances today.

Ageing and immune function

The functions of the immune system are:

- defence – recognition and destruction of foreign material e.g. pathogenic organisms or, less helpfully, transplanted tissue

- surveillance – recognition and destruction of abnormal host material like cancer cells
- homeostasis – removal and recycling of worn-out body components such as ageing red blood cells.

There is a marked similarity in the high burden of disease seen in old age to that seen in the very young whose immune system has not fully developed and in those adults whose immune system has been suppressed by drugs, disease or radiotherapy. As immunologic vigour decreases in the elderly, so there is increased incidence of infections, autoimmune and immune complex diseases, and cancer. There is general agreement that immunocompetence declines with age but details of the mechanisms involved in this loss are unclear and largely beyond the scope of this book (reviewed by Kay, 1985; Chandra, 1985).

Delayed-type hypersensitivity (DTH) responses are generally reported to be reduced in the elderly. If an antigen such as tuberculin is injected into the skin this results in an inflammatory response which in the case of tuberculin is called the Mantoux reaction. The response occurs some hours after the injection of the antigen, and hence is called a delayed-type response. Such DTH responses are a measure of the functioning of the cell-mediated arm of the immune system that is involved in graft rejection, resistance to a number of pathogens (like those that cause tuberculosis, leprosy and smallpox), resisting parasitic organisms (like the one that causes toxoplasmosis) and tumour immunosurveillance.

The age-related changes in the humoral or antibody arm of the immune system seem to be generally less than those in the cell-mediated arm; these changes are generally consistent with a deterioration in the regulation of antibody production. There are elevated levels of autoantibodies (antibodies against the body's own tissues) that are responsible for autoimmune diseases like pernicious anaemia. There may be decreased ability to produce antibodies in response to antigens, elevated levels of immune complexes (due to excess antibody production and consequent failure of antibody-antigen complexes to precipitate), and benign, antibody-producing tumours.

Changes in the skin and the mucous membranes of the gut, respiratory tract and urinary tract in the elderly may decrease the efficiency of these as barriers to infection. Changes in the secretion of mucous, ciliary movement and mechanical functioning in the gastrointestinal, respiratory and urinary tracts may all contribute to increased risk of infection and disease.

There is ample evidence (reviewed by Chandra, 1993) that malnutrition also has profound deleterious effects upon the immune system. Some of the likely effects of malnutrition upon the immune system are listed in Table 3.1. DTH responses are, once again, markedly depressed in malnutrition. Secretion of immunoglobulin A (IgA), the antibody fraction that protects mucosal surfaces, is depressed and the ability of phagocytic white cells to kill ingested bacteria is reduced in malnutrition. Thus it is quite possible that some of the decline in immunocompetence manifested in the elderly may be related to the high levels of suboptimal nutrition that may occur in some elderly populations. It is inevitable that malnutrition will compound with the effects of ageing in

Table 3.1 Some effects of malnutrition upon immunity and infection risk. Several of the conclusions are based upon studies in Third World children. Main data sources: Tomkins and Watson (1989); Chandra (1993)

1	Gastric acidity may be reduced predisposing to gastrointestinal infections
2	The effectiveness of mucosal surfaces as barriers to infection may be reduced by general malnutrition or by several micronutrient deficiencies, e.g. in vitamin A deficiency, there is reduced glycoprotein production and mucus secretion and this forms a protective layer over some mucosal surfaces
3	Wounds heal more slowly and are thus more likely to become infected
4	There is reduced secretion of IgA, the antibody that protects mucosal surfaces
5	Delayed-type hypersensitivity responses (i.e. cell-mediated immune responses) are depressed even in moderate malnutrition
6	The ability of phagocytes to kill ingested bacteria is reduced
7	The production of circulating antibody (IgG) is relatively unaffected, although the response to immunisation may be delayed.

depressing the immune function of elderly, malnourished people. The concept of a cycle of infection and malnutrition has been well established by those investigating the health of malnourished children in poorer countries; malnutrition predisposes to infection – infection worsens or precipitates malnutrition and a dangerous positive feedback cycle is established:

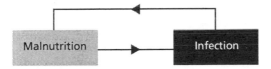

It seems reasonable to propose that a similar cycle would operate in elderly, malnourished people.

Biochemical and other indicators of nutritional deficiency have been found to be associated with reduced responses in immune function tests in disease-free, elderly people. Nutritional supplements given to these elderly subjects were associated with improvements in both the measures of nutritional status and the measures of immunocompetence (Chandra, 1985). In a more recent study, Chandra (1992) randomly assigned 96 free-living elderly people to receive either a micronutrient supplement or a placebo. After a year, several measures of immune function were higher in the supplemented group than in the controls and the supplemented group had less than half the number of days affected by infective illness as the controls. Woo et al. (1994) showed that nutritional supplements given to elderly people recovering from chest infections were effective in helping them to recover from their illness. Various measures of wellbeing and measures of nutritional status were higher in the supplemented group than in the controls.

Trauma, whether surgical or accidental, also has an immunosuppressive effect and the degree of immunosuppression is proportional to the amount of trauma (Lennard and Browell, 1993). Thus elderly and malnourished surgical patients or accident victims would be triply impaired, with likely results being, higher mortality, higher levels of general and wound infections, slower rates of healing and recovery, increased duration of hospital stay and increased costs of treatment.

Conclusions

- Maintaining nutritional status in the elderly may ameliorate some of the observed deterioration in immune function that is associated with ageing; malnutrition may be one factor in producing this age-associated decline in immune function. Malnutrition in the elderly will certainly compound with these age-related changes and depress immunocompetence still further.
- In elderly, surgical and trauma patients, particular attention should be given to monitoring and maintaining nutritional status. In those elderly people undergoing major elective surgery, nutritional assessment and corrective measures prior to surgery may be cost effective as well as being beneficial to the patient.
- Particular care needs to be taken to ensure the microbiological safety of food intended for elderly people especially the frail elderly – this is discussed in Chapter 7.

The ageing skeleton and osteoporosis

The nature of bone

Approximately 50% of the weight of bone is made up of an organic matrix containing large amounts of the protein collagen. Deposited upon this organic matrix is a crystalline mineral material that gives the bone its mechanical strength. This mineral matter is called hydroxyapatite and it is a complex calcium phosphate compound. There are two types of mature bone. 80% is cortical or compact bone found on the outside of bones. The remaining 20% is trabecular bone, which has a honeycomb structure with bone marrow filling the spaces; it is found in the centre of bones such as the pelvis, vertebrae and the ends of the long bones.

Bone is not a fixed inert material, but rather a living and constantly changing structure. Bones are continually being remodelled by cells that synthesise new bone (osteoblasts) and cells that reabsorb bone and cartilage (osteoclasts). Thus if a bone's weight remains constant this is the result of a dynamic equilibrium, a balance between bone synthesis and breakdown.

Changes in skeletal weight with age

During childhood, the total weight of the skeleton increases as the body and bones grow. The skeleton reaches its peak weight (peak bone mass, PBM) in early adulthood, between 25 and 35 years of age. The newborn baby has around 25–30 g of calcium in its body, almost all of it contained within the bone mineral and by the time the PBM is reached this skeletal calcium content has risen to well over 1 kg. After the PBM has been reached, there is a gradual loss of bone mass with age. Both organic matrix and mineral matter are lost; the bone becomes thinner, its mechanical strength is reduced and it becomes increasingly prone to fracture even when subjected to relatively minor trauma. This thinning of the bones and consequent increase in fracture risk is called osteoporosis. In men and premenopausal women this loss of bone is relatively slow, in the order of 0.3–0.4% of bone lost per year. In women, however, there is a marked acceleration in this rate of bone loss at the time of the menopause. For a few years after the start of the menopause rates of bone loss may be as much as ten times those seen in men and premenopausal women (see Figure 3.2).

The prevalence and costs of osteoporosis

Osteoporotic fractures of the vertebrae, wrist and especially the neck of the femur (hip fracture) are considered to be a major public health problem in many industrialised countries, including the UK and USA. In the UK, there are over 50,000 hip fractures each year and a significant proportion of those affected die within a few months of the initial fracture (12–20%) whilst many more never regain full mobility after the initial fracture. Up to 20,000 deaths each year may occur as a consequence of hip fracture or the associated surgery. In 1993 (NOS, 1993) it was estimated that osteoporosis patients were occupying almost a third of hospital orthopaedic beds and costing the UK National Health Service over £600 million ($900 million) per annum.

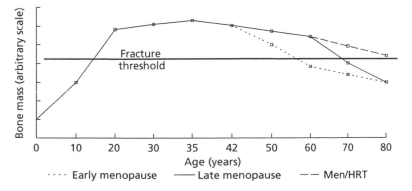

Figure 3.2 Graphical representation of changes in bone mass throughout life

Osteoporosis – who is at risk?

From the above discussion, there are two very clear but unalterable risk factors for osteoporosis; being female and being elderly. Other known or putative risk factors for osteoporosis are listed in Table 3.2. As people get older, their bone mass declines, the probability of their skeletal mass falling below the fracture threshold increases and thus also the probability of osteoporotic fracture. Accelerated rate of bone loss at the menopause means that women are likely to reach the fracture threshold earlier than men (see Figure 3.2). The fracture threshold is the skeletal mass or density at which bones become liable to fracture in response to even relatively minor traumas, like a fall from the standing position.

Table 3.2 Factors associated with increased risk of osteoporosis. Data source: Webb (1995)

Old age; risk of osteoporosis increases with age and accelerates in women when they reach the menopause

Being female; rates are higher in women than men in Western Europe and North America

Being white; there are distinct racial differences in bone density and considerable genetic variations within races

Lack of sex hormones; factors which reduce sex hormone secretion (e.g. early menopause or ovarian removal) increase risk and hormone replacement therapy reduces risk

Never having borne a child

A sedentary lifestyle

Smoking

High alcohol consumption

Being small or underweight

Inadequate calcium intake in childhood?

High consumption of carbonated, cola drinks?

Being an omnivore; vegetarians have lower rates of osteoporosis

Figure 3.3 shows the age and sex distribution of cases of hip fracture in one region of England. Most of the hip fractures in this region occurred in people over the age of 55 years. In a prospective study of 1400 elderly British people, Wickham *et al.* (1989) found that incidence of hip fracture was four times higher in women over 85 years compared to women in the 65–74 year age band. Figure 3.3 indicates that up to the age of 54 years hip fractures in males make up a bigger proportion of all fractures than those recorded in females. In the older age groups, however, fractures in women make up a far greater proportion of the total than those in older men (18.5% of total in men over 55 years compared to 75.7% of total in women over 55 years). In their prospective study, referred to above, Wickham *et al.* recorded no fractures in the men under 75 years in their sample and the incidence in the over 85s was twice as high in females as males. Spector *et al.* (1990) found a female to male ratio of 4:1 in the age-specific incidence of hip fracture in the UK.

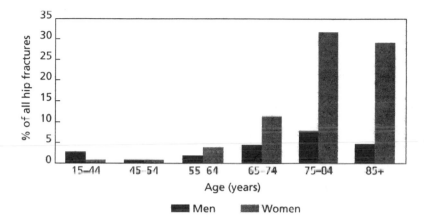

Figure 3.3 Age distribution of hip fractures in the Trent region of England 1989/1990. Data source: Kanis (1993)

Acceleration in the rate of bone loss after the start of the menopause in women is due to failing oestrogen supplies from the ageing ovary. Conditions that are associated with oestrogen deficiency in younger women also lead to reduced bone density and a consequent increase in fracture risk (e.g. early menopause, oophorectomy, amenorrhea due to low body weight, as seen in anorexia nervosa). Hyposecretion of sex hormones in men leads to a similar reduction in bone density.

Rates of osteoporotic fracture have undoubtedly increased very substantially over the last 50 years in many industrialised countries. Part of this increase is an inevitable consequence of the growth in the elderly, particularly elderly female, population. There has also, however, been an increase in the age specific fracture rates, that is there have been substantial increases in fracture rates over and above those which can be accounted for simply by the ageing of the population (Spector *et al.*, 1990). Likewise, wide variations in rates of osteoporotic fracture, even within western industrial countries, cannot be accounted for solely by differences in the proportions of elderly people. This suggests that environmental or lifestyle variations may have a considerable influence upon the risk of osteoporosis and thus that changes in lifestyle factors should have the potential to reduce fracture risk.

There are essentially three approaches that could potentially contribute to reducing the risk of osteoporosis:

- Measures aimed at increasing the PBM; this increases the amount of bone that can be lost in later life before the fracture threshold is reached. Since such measures would be directed at younger people they are outside the scope of this book.

- Attempting to slow down the rate of bone loss in older people, particularly in postmenopausal women so that it takes longer to reach fracture threshold from any given PBM.
- Reducing the risk of bones being subjected to the traumas that cause them to fracture. Fractures of the hip usually occur after a fall and so high susceptibility to falling contributes towards the increased fracture risk in the elderly. This issue is only peripherally addressed in this book but Cummings *et al.* (1985) suggest that in the already osteoporotic adult, reducing the tendency to fall may offer the greatest potential for reducing the risk of fractures. Earlier in the chapter it was suggested that reduced muscle strength may be an important factor in the propensity of some elderly people to fall; measures to improve muscle strength may reduce the risk of falling.

Slowing bone loss in elderly adults

There is compelling evidence that the administration of oestrogen (hormone replacement therapy, HRT) to menopausal women prevents or reduces the postmenopausal acceleration in rate of bone loss and reduces the risk of osteoporotic fracture. This treatment is widely accepted as being effective in the prevention of osteoporosis. The controversy about HRT concerns whether the benefits of the treatment are sufficient to outweigh any possible risks such as increased risk of uterine or perhaps even breast cancer.

The increasingly sedentary lifestyle of many people in industrialised countries is generally believed to be a contributory factor in the increased prevalence of osteoporosis. *The Allied Dunbar National Fitness Survey* (1992) and *The Health Survey for England* 1991 (White *et al.*, 1993) revealed very low levels of fitness and activity in many British adults and particularly in women – 50% of women aged 65–74 years did not have sufficient strength in their thigh muscles to stand from a chair without using their arms (see Chapter 4 for discussion of activity levels in the elderly). Activity is known to increase bone density, whilst immobilisation leads to a loss of bone mass. Athletes have higher bone densities than the population at large and increases in bone density are greatest in those parts of the skeleton subjected to the most stress, such as the racket arm of tennis players. Patients undergoing complete bed rest lose about 1% of their stable, cortical bone in a month and 1–2% of their more labile trabecular bone in a week. Increased activity in childhood and early adulthood increases the PBM and maintaining activity in middle-aged and elderly people slows down the rate of bone loss. In their sample of 1400 elderly British people, Wickham *et al.* (1989) found that risk of hip fracture was reduced in those people with higher levels of outdoor physical activity. Several studies have shown that participation in regular, sustained programmes of exercise can lead to measurable increases in bone density in postmenopausal women (e.g. Chow *et al.*, 1987).

Being underweight is associated with a higher risk of osteoporotic fracture and, in the elderly, this is often as a result of low lean body mass caused by inactivity; correcting the association between osteoporotic risk and inactivity for body mass may thus lead to underestimation of the strength of this association. More active and fitter elderly people may also be less prone to osteoporotic fracture because they are better co-ordinated and stronger and therefore less prone to falling or less liable to injury if they do fall.

Many studies have suggested that cigarette smoking is associated with reduced bone density and with increased fracture risk (Cummings *et al.*, 1985). In their sample of elderly British people, Wickham *et al.* (1989) reported a strong association between cigarette smoking and risk of hip fracture. Smoking is associated with:

- lower body weight
- reduced physical activity
- early menopause
- reduced blood oestrogen concentration (even in women receiving HRT).

These are all known associates of high fracture risk (the prevalence of smoking amongst elderly people is discussed in Chapter 4).

The role of strictly dietary factors in the aetiology of osteoporosis remains a controversial one. Two observations are, however, generally accepted.

High alcohol consumption is a risk factor for osteoporosis. Heavy drinking is associated with extensive bone loss even in relatively young adults (Smith, 1987). High alcohol consumption might also be expected to increase the risk of falling. This would be just one of many reasons for recommending moderation of alcohol intake in young or elderly people.

A vegetarian lifestyle is associated with higher bone density and reduced risk of osteoporosis (e.g. Marsh *et al.*, 1988). The interpretation of this observation is, however, complex and controversial. It is very difficult to establish to what extent, if any, this is as a result of meat avoidance *per se*. There are numerous differences in diet and lifestyle (confounding variables) between vegetarians and the general omnivorous population. Caucasian vegetarians are probably unrepresentative of the general white population in their socioeconomic status, their smoking, drinking and activity habits. There will also be many differences in the diets of vegetarians and the general omnivore population, partly as a direct consequence of meat avoidance but also as a result of heightened awareness of health issues in the selection and preparation of food.

The relationship between calcium nutrition and bone health is particularly controversial. As calcium is an essential nutrient and a major component of bone mineral it is natural that the role of calcium in the aetiology of osteoporosis should have received much attention (concisely reviewed in Webb, 1995). Likewise, the role of vitamin D needs to be considered. This vitamin is necessary for the efficient absorption of calcium from food and for the orderly deposition of bone mineral. The principal source of this vitamin for most people is by endogenous synthesis in skin when it is exposed to sunlight. Average daily intakes in the UK are only around 2–3 µg per day and this is far below the estimated requirement for those groups where endogenous synthesis cannot be relied upon because of inadequate sunlight exposure (the UK RNI for vitamin D is 10 µg per day for elderly, housebound people). To regularly and reliably achieve an intake of 10 µg per day requires the use of supplements.

There is little evidence that normal variation in dietary calcium intake has any major effect on bone density in adults (Smith, 1987; Cummings *et al.*,

1986). International comparisons often show that rates of osteoporosis are high in populations with high calcium intakes and low in those with low calcium intakes (Webb, 1995). Wickham *et al.* (1989) found no relationship between dietary calcium intake and risk of osteoporotic fracture in their sample of elderly adults.

There is nonetheless a strong case for ensuring adequacy of calcium and vitamin D in the elderly. Elderly housebound people may be at greatly increased risk of osteomalacia (loss of bone mineral due to vitamin D deficiency). In young, healthy British adults (18–65 years), plasma 25–hydroxycholecalciferol

Table 3.3 Food sources of calcium and vitamin D

Dietary standard (65+ years)	Calcium	Vitamin D
	RNI – UK	RNI – UK
	700 mg	10 µg
	RDA – US	RDA – US
	800 mg	5 µg

Note that, in practice, it is not possible to obtain the RNI for vitamin D from a normal diet.

	% of the UK RNI provided by typical food portions	
	Calcium	Vitamin D
195 g whole milk* (unsupplemented)	32	0.3–0.6
1 egg (60 g)	5	12
5 g butter	Tr	0.4
5 g margarine	0	4
40 g cheddar cheese	41	1
90 g fried lamb liver	2	5
85 g canned sardines (with bones)	56	51
80 g peeled prawns	17	Tr
5 g cod liver oil	Tr	105
20 g almonds	7	0
1 slice wholemeal bread	3	Tr
95 g broccoli	10	0

*Skimming of milk (fat removal) does not affect the calcium content of milk but all of the vitamin D is in the fat fraction. Tr = trace

levels (25OHD), a good indicator of vitamin D status, range from 15–35 ng/ml in summer to 8–18 ng/ml in winter; COMA (1991) considered these values to be satisfactory and set no Dietary Reference Values for vitamin D except for those confined indoors. In Britons over 75 years of age mean 25OHD levels average only 5 ng/ml and do not rise above 10 ng/ml even in high summer. COMA (1991) considered this to indicate unsatisfactory vitamin D status in many elderly Britons and they attributed this primarily to insufficient skin exposure to sunlight during the summer months. Low 25OHD levels are present in up to 40% of elderly people living in residential homes and hospitals (COMA, 1991). In the elderly, there is reduced efficiency in final activation of vitamin D in the kidney to yield the active hormone 1,25-dihydroxycholecalciferol.

Chapuy et al. (1994) showed that calcium and vitamin D supplements given to institutionalised, elderly women in France substantially reduced risk of hip and other fractures over a three year period. High serum parathyroid levels would be expected in vitamin D deficiency and some of their sample had raised parathyroid levels and other indications of low vitamin D status (low serum 25-hydroxycholecalciferol concentrations). The treatment lowered serum parathyroid hormone levels (levels rose in the placebo group) and high parathyroid hormone levels were associated with lowered bone density measurements. These results suggest that the supplements were effective because they corrected existing deficiencies and thus that such deficiencies are a significant contributing factor to the normal high fracture rates in this group. Table 3.3 shows the dietary standards for calcium and vitamin D in the elderly and indicates the value of some common foods as sources of these nutrients.

Higher exposure to sunlight, and thus better vitamin D status, could be a contributory factor to the protective effect of exercise on fracture risk in the elderly, that is in the negative association between outdoor physical activity and fracture risk recorded by Wickham et al. (1989) as discussed earlier. A recent expert report in the UK (CWT, 1995) recommended that architects designing residential accommodation for older people should take particular account of the need of residents for regular exposure to sunlight. They suggested the provision of sheltered alcoves on the south side of buildings and well-paved pathways with hand rails and no steps.

Bone health in ethnic minorities

There are racial differences in bone density and risk of osteoporosis. In general, persons of European and Asian origin have bones that are less dense than people of African origin. In the United States white women are much more likely to experience osteoporotic fractures than black women.

Given the importance currently attached to achieving a high peak bone mass in early adulthood one might speculate that there will in the future be high rates of osteoporotic fracture amongst British Asian women who have spent their childhood in the UK. In the 1960s and 1970s there were mini epidemics of rickets amongst Asian children and women in the UK (e.g. see Robertson et al., 1982). It will still be some years before there are large numbers of elderly British Asian women who spent their childhoods in Britain.

Age-dependent changes in disease risk factors

Aims and scope of the chapter

Risk factors in disease causation

Some specific risk factors:

- overweight and underweight

- reduced glucose tolerance

- inactivity

- high blood pressure

- high plasma/serum cholesterol

- alcohol consumption

- cigarette smoking

A summary of current nutrition education guidelines – are they suitable for older adults?

Aims and scope of the chapter

In recent years nutrition research has been dominated by studies that seek to:

- measure the effect of diet on certain risk factors for disease
- clarify the aetiological pathways that link diet, risk factors and disease.

Attempts to alter risk factors and thus reduce disease risk are key elements in many programmes for nutrition education, preventive medicine and health promotion. This chapter has four broad aims:

- to describe some of the age-related changes that occur in important risk factors
- to try to identify the reasons for these age-related changes and to decide how much of this age-related change is an inevitable consequence of ageing
- to consider whether dietary and other measures designed to reduce risk factors in younger people are appropriate and likely to produce holistic benefit in older people

- where appropriate, to try to define some broad, low risk strategies that, at the population level, are likely to contribute to a reduction in disease by affecting risk factors.

Note that much of the data on age-related changes in risk factors may not be entirely representative because it has been obtained solely from elderly people still living in their own homes and so has excluded the large minority of elderly people living in residential care accommodation. There are also some apparent ethnic differences in risk factor levels and significance, several of which are highlighted.

The dietary management of those with established disease (e.g. diabetes) or those with levels of risk factors that are frankly pathological (e.g. hyperlipidaemia) is discussed in Chapter 8.

Risk factors in disease causation

Certain measured parameters and lifestyle characteristics partially predict an individual's likelihood of suffering from or dying of a particular disease or simply of dying prematurely.

- An elevated serum cholesterol concentration is widely accepted as indicating an increased risk of developing coronary heart disease
- High blood pressure is associated with increased risk of renal failure, heart disease and stroke
- Being overweight is associated with increased likelihood of developing maturity onset, or non-insulin-dependent, diabetes mellitus (NIDDM).

In many cases these risk markers are thought to be causally linked to the development of the associated disease, i.e. they are not just markers for those at risk but are true risk factors that directly contribute to the development of the disease. Thus a high serum cholesterol level is generally believed to accelerate the atherosclerotic changes in arteries that lead to increased risk of coronary heart disease. Such an assumption of cause and effect would suggest that altering the risk factor (lowering serum cholesterol), should also reduce the risk of the disease, provided such changes occur before there is irreversible damage. Much current health promotion, nutrition education and preventive medicine is based upon such assumptions. Diet is considered to be a key element in this risk factor reduction. Of course, the proviso that lowering risk factors is only likely to work if damage is not already irreversible must apply particularly to older people. In some cases the evidence that intervention, including dietary change, has net beneficial effects is controversial even in younger people and the case for intervention in older people will often be weaker still.

Differentiating between association and causation

Association between a risk factor/lifestyle variable and a disease does not necessarily mean that there is a cause and effect relationship. It is quite probable that the statistical link between a risk marker and a disease may have arisen because both are associated with a third, confounding variable. For example, even though alcohol may not directly contribute to causing lung cancer, a statistical association between alcohol consumption and lung cancer might arise if heavy drinkers also tend to be heavy smokers. To take a more topical example, there is an inverse relationship between a population's intake of dietary fibre and the mortality rate for bowel cancer, so perhaps dietary fibre directly protects against bowel cancer? There is, however, also a positive association between bowel cancer and fat intake and an inverse relationship between the fat and fibre contents of population diets (i.e. high fat diets tend to be low in fibre and vice versa). Thus an alternative explanation could be that high fat intake causes bowel cancer and that the apparent protective effect of fibre is merely an artefact due to the inverse relationship between fat and fibre intakes.

Epidemiologists almost always try to identify and allow for the effects of confounding variables when trying to establish a causative link between a risk marker and a disease. There is, however, no statistical magic wand that unerringly and accurately corrects for all confounding variables; it is a matter of judgement what the likely confounders are and the process of correction itself may be imprecise, particularly if there is imprecise or limited measurement of the confounding variable (Leon, 1990).

Age as a confounding variable

Age is a confounding variable in many epidemiological studies because the incidence of many diseases increases with age. Age can usually be precisely measured and therefore age correction should be reliable. Likewise, in many experimental studies subjects will be age-matched. However, anything that changes as a result of ageing will predict mortality in the elderly and be associated with diseases of ageing even when correction for chronological age is made (Burr, 1985). Chronological age is an imperfect indicator of physiological ageing and some age-related changes in physiological/biochemical parameters may be much better indicators of the subjects' true biological age. They may thus be ideal predictors of the likelihood of developing age-related disease without being directly involved in their causation. To take a hypothetical example, loss of hair pigment is likely to be associated with increased risk of dying of several of the age-related diseases but there is no reason to suspect that this association is causative. Even if one corrected this association for chronological age, then if greying of the hair is an indicator of age-related physiological deterioration, it might still be a significant predictor of mortality risk.

Risk factor reduction

Once it has been accepted that a risk factor is causally linked to the development of a particular disease or diseases, then health promotion/nutrition education aimed at reducing the risk factor and thus prevention of the disease may be considered appropriate. There are essentially two approaches to risk reduction.

- **The population approach** – advice is directed at the whole population, or large sections of it, with the aim of reducing average population exposure to the risk.
- **The individual approach** – efforts are made to identify those most at risk from the risk factor and intervention is targeted specifically at these 'high risk' individuals.

If one takes the example of a programme aimed at lowering serum cholesterol in order to reduce morbidity and mortality from coronary heart disease, then one could choose either of the following options.

- Take the population approach, direct the message at the whole adult population; if successful this would then be expected to lower average serum cholesterol concentrations and shift the whole population distribution of serum cholesterol concentrations downwards.
- Alternatively, one could seek to identify those with highly elevated serum cholesterol concentrations and thus most at risk from coronary heart disease. The cholesterol-lowering messages could then be targeted much more specifically at these high risk individuals.

Much health promotion/nutrition education in the UK, has tended to use the population approach. If one is seeking to make significant impact upon population mortality/morbidity from a disease as in the *Health of the Nation* targets (DH, 1992b), the population approach appears to offer the greatest probability of success. If we return to the earlier serum cholesterol example, there are relatively few younger adults with highly elevated serum cholesterol concentrations (say over 7.8 mmol/l) and so even a substantial reduction of risk in this group will do little to affect population mortality from coronary heart disease. There are many more young and middle-aged adults (the majority of the population) who have serum cholesterol concentrations that are regarded as slightly or moderately elevated (say 5.2–7.8 mmol/l). Even a small reduction in individual risks for this very large group will have a significant effect upon total population mortality. Some other advantages of the population approach are discussed below.

- Because the changes are directed at everyone the promoted behaviour may become the norm and so some consequent social and economic changes may make it easier for any individual to change. If advice to reduce fat and saturated fat intake is directed at the whole population, this increases the incentive for food manufacturers and distributors to develop and market products that are low in fat and/or saturated fat (e.g.

    low-fat spreads
    margarines and oils that are low in saturated fat
    lower fat milks
    and, low-fat processed foods)

Adoption of a low-fat diet is facilitated by the ready availability of such foods and low-fat choices may become to be perceived as the norm.

- The population approach also removes the need to identify the high risk subjects and the need to mark them out as 'victims' of a particular condition. On the other hand, an individual approach to cholesterol-lowering may be seen to require a universal screening programme to identify those above some arbitrary cut-off point for serum cholesterol; if screening is not universal then some high risk individuals may not be identified.
- Once identified by screening, high risk individuals would probably feel much more threatened by their 'high risk' classification and change might be more difficult for them to implement because the changes in product availability and social norms discussed above would be unlikely to occur.

There are also disadvantages to the population, as follows.

- The population approach requires mass change and, for many, that change will offer only a small reduction in individual risk and thus the motivation to change may be greatly reduced.
- If mass change is induced, then there is increased likelihood that some currently 'low risk' individuals may be harmed by the change. For example, there is evidence that a very low serum cholesterol concentration (less than 4.2 mmol/l) may be associated with an increase in total mortality (Neaton *et al.*, 1992; Jacobs *et al.*, 1992). If there really is a causal association between low serum cholesterol and some diseases, then the population approach to cholesterol-lowering will have an adverse effect on those people with already very low serum cholesterol concentrations and tend to push some other people into this very low category.
- The evidence for the benefits of many of the current nutrition education guidelines are strongest in young and middle-aged adults (some might say particularly young and middle-aged men). Is all of this advice equally appropriate for the elderly and very elderly? If not then the population approach to nutrition education may create norms of behaviour and even changes in the range and pricing of foods that are not to the advantage of this large minority of the adult population. Similarly, if there are ethnic differences in the significance of some risk factors then these changes may not be to the advantage of some ethnic minority groups.
- The population approach also risks creating an unhealthy preoccupation with death and disease in the whole population (McCormick and Skrabanek, 1988). Even people at very low risk of coronary heart disease may be made extremely fearful of this condition. This would be particularly true if health promotion focused upon the negative aspects of not accepting the message, that is if it used fear of death and disease and the threat of social isolation as the primary levers for effecting dietary or other behaviour change.
- The population approach may lead to those with some diseases being blamed for their condition; you have heart disease because you smoke/eat badly/do not take enough exercise. It may perhaps be used by doctors and politicians to justify the withholding of expensive treatments.

Some specific risk factors

In this section we have selected some well-established disease risk factors for particular discussion. In some cases, the distinction between the general physiological effects of ageing discussed in Chapter 3 and the effects of ageing upon disease risk factors is somewhat artificial. Nevertheless, given the prominence attached to risk factors in nutrition education and research, we feel that they warrant more specific discussion.

Overweight and underweight

Numerous diseases and problems are associated with overweight and obesity:

- cardiovascular disease
- maturity onset diabetes
- hypertension
- hernia
- increased surgical risk
- higher accident rate
- gall bladder disease
- gout
- arthritis
- reduced mobility.

Body Mass Index (BMI) is used as an anthropometric indicator of an individual's level of fatness (see Chapter 6):

$$\text{Body Mass Index} = \frac{\text{weight in kilograms}}{(\text{height in metres})^2}$$

The assumption is that increasing weight at any given height reflects increasing amounts of stored fat. The following ranges are usually used:

<20 kg/m²	underweight
20–25 kg/m²	ideal range
25–30 kg/m²	overweight
30+ kg/m²	obese

In elderly people, particularly elderly women, loss of bone and lean tissue may mean that the amount of body fat is much higher than the BMI would suggest.

Table 4.1 shows the BMIs recorded from a representative sample of English adults. Values in young, but mature, adults (25–34 years) are compared with those found in the three oldest age bands used in this survey. This survey shows that in English adults levels of overweight and obesity increase with age, peak in late middle-age and then start to decline. Loss of bone mass and lean tissue in old age means that the threshold values used may slightly understate the degree of adiposity of older adults. The combined levels of overweight and obesity in elderly English adults is extremely high: around 60% of all men and

Table 4.1 Comparison of mean and percentage distribution of BMIs in selected age groups of a representative sample of English adults. Data source: White et al. (1993)

Age	BMI (kg/m²)				
	Mean	<20	20–25	25–30	30+
Male					
All 16+ years	25.6	6	42	40	13
25–34 years	24.9	5	52	35	8
55–64 years	26.9	4	29	48	19
65–74 years	26.4	3	37	45	14
75+ years	25.7	8	38	47	7
Female					
All 16+ years	25.4	9	47	29	16
25–34 years	24.2	14	54	19	12
55–64 years	27.3	4	37	34	25
65–74 years	26.3	6	34	41	19
75+ years	25.9	7	41	36	16

women aged 65–74 years are either overweight or obese. Note, however, that levels of overweight and obesity are lower in the over 75s and, in men, the prevalence of underweight is higher than the prevalence of obesity.

Dietary and lifestyle practices that assist in 'normalising' body weight would thus seem to be of relevance to the majority of the elderly population. Inactivity is almost certainly important in precipitating increases in the rates of overweight and obesity in populations. Average energy intakes have been falling since the 1950s in Britain and yet the rates of overweight and obesity have been increasing. Energy expenditure has been declining due to reduced requirements for physical activity brought about by automation in the work-place, home and garden and by increased reliance upon vehicle transportation. This has not been completely offset by decreases in energy intake. There are good grounds for recommending increased levels of activity in all age groups and this should also contribute to a reduced prevalence of overweight and obesity.

The energy density of the diet is the number of calories per unit weight of food. Reducing the energy density of the diet is seen as an important dietary goal (e.g. NACNE, 1983). It is reasoned that a bulkier diet should decrease the likelihood of overconsumption and thus should assist in weight control. The energy density of diets can be reduced by replacing some of the dietary fat with starchy and fibre-rich foods. Refined sugars and alcohol contribute high-ly palatable calories to the diet but few nutrients and may also raise the energy density of the diet and encourage overconsumption.

At the population level
- Increased activity levels in younger people and maintenance of physical activity levels in the elderly should contribute to reducing the levels of overweight and obesity in addition to its other health benefits.

- A bulkier diet with fewer calories per unit weight of food may contribute to improved body weight control. Reduced energy density of the diet can be achieved by reducing the amounts of fat and extrinsic sugars in the diet and replacing them with starchy and fibre-rich foods.

In young and middle-aged men and women, there is overwhelming evidence that overweight, and particularly obesity, are associated with excess morbidity and reduced life expectancy. However, this conclusion becomes much less secure in older people. As seen in Table 4.1, the prevalence of overweight and obesity also starts to decline in late middle-age and a significant minority of the over 75s are underweight. Exton-Smith (1988) suggested that in the elderly, high body weight is associated with increased life expectancy rather than, as in young and middle-aged people, with reduced life expectancy. Lehmann (1991), in a review of nutrition in old age concluded that 'being underweight is numerically and prognostically of far greater importance than obesity in most groups of elderly people studied'. She suggests that, in the elderly, being moderately overweight is not associated with any excess mortality risk whereas underweight is associated with:

- increased mortality, whether measured in well elderly people living at home, or patients admitted to hospital
- increased risk of hip fracture
- increased risk of infections
- increased risk of specific nutrient deficiencies.

Being underweight and having low reserves of energy and nutrients may leave elderly people less able to survive periods of illness, injury, or indeed any circumstances that adversely affect health and nutritional status.

The combined effects of low body weight, reduced lean tissue to fat ratio and extreme inactivity may also reduce the maintenance energy requirements of these elderly individuals very substantially and threaten their ability to obtain adequate intakes of the other essential nutrients. Energy rich, but nutrient depleted foods (i.e. foods with low nutrient density, that is, low amounts of nutrient per calorie) will further depress the intakes of essential nutrients. Foods that contribute to this include sugary foods and drinks, alcoholic drinks, fats and oils (see Chapter 5).

At least in the short term, low body weight rather than high body weight may be the better predictor of mortality in the elderly. Two studies, described below, illustrate this point.

Campbell et al. (1990)

In a study of 750 New Zealanders over the age of 70 years, Campbell found that anthropometric indicators of low body weight, low body fat stores and particularly low muscle bulk were associated with an increased risk of death in the four years following measurement. In contrast, neither those with a high body mass index (above the 90th percentile) nor those with high skinfold triceps thickness (a measure of body fat stores – see Chapter 6) had any increased risk of death over this period.

Mattila *et al.* (1986)

In a study with very elderly (over 85 years), Finnish people, Mattila found a progressive increase in the five year survival rate as BMI increased. The highest survival rate was in those people with BMIs in excess of 28 kg/m^2. They cautioned against the use of body weight reduction in very elderly people.

Of course, these studies were of relatively short duration, and low body weights and loss of fat and protein stores may be early indicators of existing ill health. Also, as with any predictor of premature mortality, one would expect the predictive value of obesity to decline in elderly subjects. There may well be a general tendency for elderly people to lose weight at the end of their lives and thus weight loss may be a physiological indicator of ageing. Nevertheless, such findings have now been reported by several different research groups and they suggest the need to exercise caution before prescribing reducing diets to very elderly subjects.

An expert working party on the nutrition of elderly people (COMA, 1992) recommended that there should be more research aimed at clarifying the prognostic significance of BMI in the elderly. They discuss data from a 10-year cohort study of elderly people (65–74 years) which found that the relationship between mortality and BMI was U-shaped with a tendency for mortality to rise at the extremes of the range (very low or very high BMI). In men this U-curve was markedly skewed with the lowest mortality recorded in men with BMIs in the 60th to 84th percentile. There were some sex differences in the relationship between BMI and subsequent mortality, with the lowest mortality in women seen in those with BMIs in the middle of the range i.e. between the 40th and 59th percentile. Perhaps these sex differences are related to the shorter life expectancies of men and might suggest that the low-point of mortality tends to skew towards higher BMI towards the end of life.

In Chapter 8, there is some discussion of the treatment of obesity in the elderly, including the difficult issue of when treatment should be instigated.

There is a substantial and growing body of evidence which suggests that a high waist:hip ratio is an important determinant of the health risks of obesity. Obesity with a typical male pattern of fat distribution, a high waist:hip ratio, carries a greater risk than that associated with a low waist:hip ratio, a typical female pattern of distribution. It seems that much of the health risks of obesity are associated with fat deposited in the abdominal cavity (concisely reviewed by Seidell, 1992). Table 4.2 shows how waist:hip ratio increases with age in both sexes; not only are overweight and obesity more prevalent in older adults but it is also associated with a higher waist:hip ratio than in younger people. Standards and optimal ranges for waist:hip ratio are still very tentative but upper desirable limits of 1.0 or 0.95 have been suggested for men and 0.8 for women; a substantial majority of older women are above this proposed target and a majority of older men above 0.95. The prognostic significance of waist:hip ratio in the elderly is an area that has not yet received much specific attention and the appropriateness of the tentative optimal ranges given above has not been established.

Table 4.2 A comparison of waist:hip ratios in selected age groups from a representative sample of English adults. Data source: White *et al.* (1993)

Age	Mean	Waist:hip ratio (% of population sector shown) Band				
		1	2	3	4	5
Male						
All 16+ years	0.901	20	20	20	20	20
25–34 years	0.870	33	31	19	11	5
55–64 years	0.930	9	12	24	23	32
65–74 years	0.931	10	9	21	28	32
75+ years	0.938	6	11	16	28	39
Female						
All 16+ years	0.794	20	20	20	20	20
25–34 years	0.770	33	22	22	11	12
55–64 years	0.815	7	17	20	28	27
65–74 years	0.830	6	12	15	28	39
75+ years	0.842	2	9	17	31	41

The bands are:
♂ 1: <0.844; 2: 0.844–0.887; 3: 0.887–0.920; 4: 0.920–0.958; 5: 0.958+
♀ 1: <0.739; 2: 0.739–0.772; 3: 0.772–0.802; 4: 0.802–0.847; 5: 0.847+

Reduced glucose tolerance

Maturity onset or non-insulin-dependent diabetes (NIDDM) is one of the so-called 'diseases of industrialisation'. It is prevalent in affluent countries where food is plentiful, activity levels low and where rates of overweight and obesity are high. Environmental factors like diet and lifestyle are undoubt-edly precipitating factors because it is rare in peasant communities but common amongst people from the same genetic background who have migrated to affluent countries. In the UK, people of Asian origin have five times higher rates of NIDDM than the rate in the white population (DH, 1991). In general, groups who have relatively recently adopted a 'western lifestyle' and who are adapted to life in situations where food supply is fru-gal and hard physical labour the norm, seem particularly susceptible to this form of diabetes. There is also undoubtedly a genetic element in this disease, so people inherit varying susceptibilities to NIDDM but it is precipitated by environmental factors.

NIDDM is associated with reduced life expectancy and an increased risk of disability in later years. Diabetics are more likely to suffer from coronary heart disease, to have elevated blood pressure, to go blind due to retinopathy and cataract, to lose peripheral sensation (neuropathy); to suffer from gangrene with the consequent risk of amputations and suffer from progressive loss of renal function (diabetic nephropathy).

Ageing is associated with a general deterioration in the ability to maintain glucose homeostasis which manifests as impaired tolerance to a glucose load. There is a small but measurable age-related increase in the fasting blood glucose concentration and a more substantial increase in the blood glucose concentration two hours after an oral glucose load. A large US survey suggested that around 30% of people aged 60–74 years had either impaired glucose tolerance (13%) or NIDDM (17%) (Evans and Meredith, 1989). These age-related changes occur more rapidly in some ethnic groups with consequent earlier onset of NIDDM for instance in British Asians and the native American Indian population.

An official estimate in the UK (DH, 1991) put the prevalence of diagnosed diabetics in the over 65s at about 4.5%. However, this report also suggested that true prevalence of diabetes in the whole population was probably about double the number of diagnosed cases. When one further considers that most of the undiagnosed diabetics would be concentrated in the older age groups then the true prevalence of diabetes and impaired glucose tolerance in older people in the UK may not be too far below the very high US estimate of Evans and Meredith. It is also predicted in this report that because the prevalence of diabetes increases with age and the number of very elderly people in the UK population is rising, there will be a substantial increase (around 19,000 cases) in the number of diabetics aged over 70 years during the next decade (DH, 1991).

This declining glucose tolerance in middle-aged and elderly people seems to be a consequence of 'insulin resistance', reduced tissue sensitivity to insulin coupled with a relative inadequacy of insulin secretion by the pancreas. There seems to be a strong association between insulin resistance and the amount of abdominal body fat; it is associated with overweight and obesity, particularly if there is also a high waist:hip ratio. Macnair (1994) argues that insulin resistance occurs when there is a failure to use up body stores of glycogen in physical activity and thus that inactivity is implicated in insulin resistance (inactivity also seems to be implicated in increased abdominal fat deposition). Evans and Meredith (1989) and Keen and Thomas (1988) suggest that an increase in the proportion of dietary energy that is in the form of carbohydrate results in an increased sensitivity of peripheral tissues to insulin. It is also well accepted that dietary fibre (non-starch polysaccharide) improves glucose tolerance in diabetics and non- diabetics alike (discussed in Chapter 8).

The above discussion indicates that a large minority of the elderly population of many industrialised countries is at risk from diabetes itself or from the degenerative changes associated with frank NIDDM or impaired glucose tolerance. Dietary measures or other lifestyle changes that ameliorate the symptoms of diabetes or reduce the long-term consequences of NIDDM and glucose intolerance are thus of relevance to a substantial minority of elderly people and may be relevant to many of the others whose decline in glucose tolerance could be slowed by such measures.

Evans and Meredith (1989) review evidence that age *per se* is a relatively minor determinant of the age-related deterioration in glucose tolerance; factors like increased levels of inactivity, overweight and obesity (particularly 'abdominal obesity') and a high fat, low fibre diet may be responsible for the bulk of this deterioration. They suggest that replacement of some dietary fat by starch and fibre, weight loss and increased levels of activity and fitness improve glucose tolerance in the elderly. Initiating these changes earlier in life is likely to be even more effective by preventing or reducing the age-related deterioration in glucose tolerance. The role of diet in the management of elderly diabetics is reviewed in Chapter 8.

Inactivity

In Chapter 3, there was a discussion of the very large decline in all aspects of fitness that is associated with ageing (aerobic capacity, strength, endurance and flexibility all decline sharply with age in adults). It was suggested that much of this decline was not as a result of ageing *per se* but was the result of declining levels of activity with age. There was also compelling evidence that even in very elderly people, some of this age-related deterioration could be reversed by appropriate training. Both the *Allied Dunbar National Fitness Survey* (1992) and *The Health Survey for England 1991* (White *et al.*, 1993) give ample evidence of the decline in the average activity levels of British adults with age.

Table 4.3 illustrates this decline in average activity levels with age. Well over a third of those aged 65–74 years, reported engaging in no activity that could be classified even as moderate in the four week period surveyed. This figure rose to around two-thirds in the over 75 year age group. This trend cannot be completely explained by declining capabilities leading to curtailed activities because the trend is well established even in early middle age.

One of the stated aims in *The Health of the Nation* is 'to develop strategies to increase physical activity' (DH, 1992). In the equivalent American document (DHHS, 1992) there are more specific targets; for example by the year 2000, no more than 22% of over 65s should fail to engage in any leisure-time physical activity. Many studies have suggested that higher levels of physical activity and fitness are associated with long-term health benefits and a number of these apparent benefits of physical activity may be greater in older people. Some examples are listed below.

- Increased activity is associated with reduced levels of osteoporotic fracture in elderly people (e.g. Wickham *et al.*, 1989).
- Increased physical activity was associated with reduced all-cause mortality in a sample of 17,000 men age 35–74 years. These benefits were not confined to younger men – there was evidence of a beneficial effect of physical activity upon life expectancy right up to 80 years (Paffenbarger *et al.*, 1986).

Table 4.3 Distribution of reported activity levels of a representative sample of English adults. All values are percentages. Data source: White et al. (1993)

Activity level		Age group (years)				
		16–34	35–44	45–64	65–74	75+
4 and 5	♂	37	24	9	2	–
	♀	22	11	8	1	–
3	♂	23	29	38	31	13
	♀	28	34	42	21	10
1 and 2	♂	31	33	33	36	27
	♀	39	48	34	35	26
0	♂	8	15	20	31	60
	♀	10	8	16	43	65

Activity levels:
4 and 5	12 or more occasions in four weeks of vigorous or mixed vigorous/moderate activity;
3	12 or more occasions of moderate activity in four weeks;
1 and 2	one to 11 occasions of at least moderate activity in four weeks;
0	no occasions of moderate or vigorous activity in four weeks.

Moderate activity means requiring an energy expenditure of 5+ kcal/min and vigorous activity 7.5+ kcal/min.

moderate activities: walking a mile at brisk or fast pace; heavy gardening work such as digging or cutting large areas of grass by hand; heavy DIY work such as knocking down walls or breaking up concrete; heavy housework such as walking with heavy loads of shopping or scrubbing/polishing floors by hand.

vigorous activities: running or jogging; playing squash; several other sporting activities if they cause the subject to breathe heavily or sweat a lot, such as aerobics, tennis, weight training or swimming

- Morris et al. (1980) reported greatly reduced risk of coronary heart disease (CHD) in middle-aged male civil servants who had reported engaging in vigorous leisure-time physical activity compared to those who had not. The rise in CHD mortality with age was much less in the active group than in the inactive group. The advantages of the voluntary exercise continued into early old age with many fewer coronary deaths and non-fatal 'episodes' in the active men in their late sixties and early seventies. Overall, their results suggested that the advantages of leisure-time exercise seemed to increase with age.
- Blair et al. (1989) found a negative association between death rate and physical fitness in a large cohort that included both men and women. In both sexes the decline in death rate with higher level of physical fitness was most pronounced in the older age groups.
- There are likely to be psychological benefits resulting from increased physical activity. These may be direct effects of the physical activity, or indirect

effects caused by the improved physical capabilities and conditioning that increased activity brings with it. There is evidence that those elderly people with the higher levels of customary physical activity also have higher morale and that higher levels of activity contribute to maintaining this morale as they get older (Bennett and Morgan, 1992).

- Older people who maintain their levels of activity and fitness, are likely to remain able to live independently and perform the activities of daily living for longer – this must maintain self-esteem and the quality of life in later years.

Social isolation and loneliness amongst elderly people is a widespread problem (see Chapter 1); being partly or wholly housebound is a major factor in this problem.

- Increased activity leads to increased energy expenditure, both directly and as a result of the associated higher lean body (muscle) mass. Low energy requirements and therefore low food intakes cause reduced intakes of other nutrients and may precipitate inadequacy (see Chapter 5).
- Several studies have indicated that exercise increases the high density lipoprotein (HDL) cholesterol concentration in blood (Macnair, 1994). HDL is the cholesterol fraction that seems to be protective against heart disease and is not readily increased by dietary means.

High blood pressure

In industrialised countries blood pressure tends to rise with age and the prevalence of hypertension increases with age. Figure 4.1 shows the relationship between age and blood pressure in a representative cross-section of English women (White et al., 1993). Average systolic and diastolic blood pressures rise through the age bands; essentially similar results were obtained for men. Many of the subjects used for Figure 4.1 were taking antihypertensive drugs. The proportion of people taking antihypertensive drugs increased very markedly with age, such that more than a third of all over 65s were taking drugs that could have affected their blood pressure. This means that Figure 4.1 probably underestimates the real rise in blood pressure with age in Britain. White et al. (1993) defined normotensives as those with a systolic blood pressure below 160 mm/Hg and a diastolic pressure below 95 mm/Hg. Figure 4.2 shows the proportion of English adults at various ages who were normotensive and not taking drugs that could have affected their blood pressure. Around three-quarters of the over 75s were either taking antihypertensive drugs or had measured blood pressures that were classified as hypertensive. In the UK, rates of hypertension are much higher amongst Afro-Caribbeans than amongst the white population and likewise black Americans are more susceptible to hypertension than white Americans. It has been suggested that people of African origin have an ethnic predisposition to hypertension due to a hypersensitivity to salt (Law et al., 1991a).

This rise in blood pressure with age, which is generally seen in industrialised countries, does not occur in many primitive rural populations and

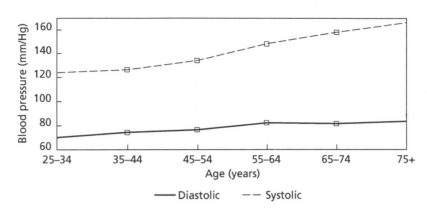

Figure 4.1 Effects of ageing on average blood pressure in English women. Data source: White *et al.* (1993)

hypertension is rare in such populations. A high population salt intake is widely thought to contribute to this age dependent rise in population blood pressure and many nutritional guidelines for industrialised countries include a recommendation to moderate salt intakes with target values of around 6 g salt per day (e.g. NRC, 1989a; NACNE, 1983). COMA (1992) concluded that this 6 g/day figure was a reasonable average for elderly Britons and recommended that current intakes be reduced to this figure. Current UK salt intake is estimated to be around 9 g/day (James *et al.*, 1987) but there is little information on how or if salt intake changes with age; the reduced taste acuity in older people discussed in Chapter 3 might increase use of salt in some older people.

High blood pressure is associated with increased risk of coronary heart disease, cerebrovascular disease (stroke), renal disease and retinal damage. In line with their predisposition to hypertension, black Americans and Afro-Caribbeans in the UK have particularly high stroke mortality.

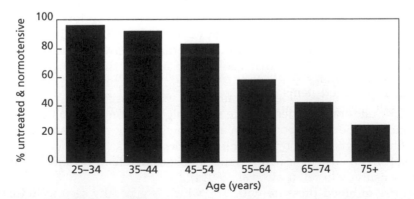

Figure 4.2 Percentage of English adults, by age, who are both normotensive and untreated. Data source: White *et al.* (1993)

Moderation of salt intake in younger people may, in the longer term, contribute to a reduction in the age-dependent rise in the average blood pressure of adults (illustrated in Figures 4.1 and 4.2) and thus contribute to a reduced incidence of hypertension in the elderly. There have also been many controlled trials of moderate salt reduction as a method of reducing blood pressure. These have generally reported some lowering of blood pressure in individuals with high initial blood pressure. There is some indication that in elderly people blood pressure may be particularly responsive to reductions in salt intake (COMA, 1992). Law *et al.* (1991b) analysed the combined results of 78 clinical trials of salt reduction upon blood pressure. They concluded that, in those trials of at least 5 weeks duration, a 3 g per day reduction in salt intake in people of 50–59 years with high blood pressure resulted in an average drop in systolic blood pressure of 7 mm/Hg and about half this reduction in diastolic blood pressure.

Table 4.4 The salt content of typical portions of some common foods. These values should be compared to the upper limit of 6 g/day recommended in the US and UK.

Major sources of dietary salt (sodium chloride) are processed foods with relatively small amounts in natural foods; discretionary salt, i.e. that added during cooking and at the table, accounts for around 15% of total UK salt intake.

1 slice wholemeal bread – 0.5 g	40 g cheddar cheese – 0.6 g
40 g Danish blue type cheese – 1.4 g	45 g All-Bran – 1.9 g
25 g cornflakes – 0.7 g	4 fish fingers – 0.9 g
85 g canned sardines – 1.5 g	80 g prawns – 3.2 g
120 g gammon steak – 6.5 g	60 g corned beef – 1.5 g
2 pork sausages (UK) – 1.5 g	small packet salted peanuts – 0.3 g
145 g canned tomato soup – 1.7 g	small packet crisps(chips) – 0.4 g
200 g baked beans – 2.4 g	60 g liver pate – 1.1 g

According to James *et al.* (1987) around three-quarters of the average UK salt intake is derived from salt added by manufacturers during the processing of foods, e.g. in cheese, bacon and meat products, bread, canned foods and ready meals. Table 4.4 gives some examples of the salt content of typical portions of some common food items. Only around 15% of total salt intake is 'discretionary salt' added directly by the consumer during home cooking and at the table. This means that cutting down on these direct uses of salt can only produce modest reductions in total salt consumption and that to cut salt intake by a third will require either changing the food selections of elderly people or for food manufacturers to use less salt in processing. Salt is a major preservative as well as a flavouring agent and so cutting down on the use of salt and other preservatives may affect the microbiological safety of food which is particularly important for the elderly who are more susceptible to foodborne pathogens and whose living conditions (e.g. relative poverty, low mobility and living alone) may make them more likely to eat stale food.

A number of other factors are known to influence blood pressure and thus affect the risk of hypertension. Obesity and high alcohol consumption are two well established risk factors for hypertension. Higher BMI was associated with higher blood pressure in both sexes in a representative survey of English adults (White *et al.*, 1993). In male drinkers, blood pressure rose with increasing alcohol consumption (but note that the blood pressure of non-drinkers was higher than that of low and moderate drinkers). Low potassium intake or high sodium:potassium ratio may also be significant factors; potassium intakes would be very dependent upon the amounts of fruits and vegetables consumed as these are major sources of dietary potassium. High calcium intakes, high levels of physical activity and physical fitness may also be protective factors that reduce the risk of hypertension.

Several dietary/lifestyle objectives (listed below), that can be justified on other grounds, would, if implemented together, almost certainly contribute to a substantial reduction in blood pressure in the elderly. They could thus be expected to reduce the heavy dependence upon antihypertensive drugs that are used to minimise the consequences of hypertension in the elderly:

- increased physical activity and physical fitness
- reduced incidence of overweight and obesity (but note the earlier discussion about old age being a possible contra-indicator for weight reduction)
- moderation of excessive alcohol consumption
- increased consumption of fruit and vegetables and thus potassium
- meeting the dietary standards for calcium intakes.

It also seems probable that substantial reductions in salt intake in the hypertensive elderly will contribute to a reduction in blood pressure, although there may be major practical difficulties in implementing this change. Elderly people who can only shop infrequently and for a variety of reasons may be unable or unwilling to prepare food from raw, unprocessed ingredients may find it particularly difficult to reduce their salt intake by a substantial amount. Declining taste acuity may tend to encourage increased use of salt in elderly people. The general population target of an average of 6 g of salt per day should also apply to the elderly (COMA, 1992).

High plasma/serum cholesterol

SIGNIFICANCE OF PLASMA CHOLESTEROL

A high plasma cholesterol concentration is predictive of an increased risk of coronary heart disease (CHD). This association between plasma cholesterol and increased risk of CHD is generally accepted to be the result of a cause and effect relationship. According to the diet-heart hypothesis (Figure 4.3), high plasma cholesterol leads to atherosclerotic changes in artery walls which are the major cause of coronary heart disease. Nutrition education guidelines aimed at reducing average plasma cholesterol concentrations are one of the key themes of health promotion in many industrialised countries. The expectation is that implementation of these cholesterol-lowering measures would lead to a fall in morbidity and mortality from CHD and other conditions associated with atherosclerosis. As these are such major causes of mortality and morbidity ultimately this would be expected to lead to improved life expectancy and/or reduced total morbidity. The following ranges for plasma total cholesterol are widely used:

less than 5.2 mmol/l	desirable
5.2–6.5 mmol/l	mildly elevated
6.5–7.8 mmol/l	moderately elevated
7.8+ mmol/l	severely elevated

There is ethnic variation in the significance of particular risk factors for CHD. British Asians have much higher rates of CHD than the white population despite their lower exposure to many of the traditional risk factors for CHD (they consume less saturated fat and cholesterol, have lower plasma cholesterol levels, smoke less and drink less alcohol according to McKeigue et al., 1985). McKeigue et al. (1991) attribute this increased risk of CHD to high prevalence of insulin resistance, abdominal obesity and diabetes. They suggest that high energy intakes and inactivity are the likely environmental causes of these metabolic disturbances.

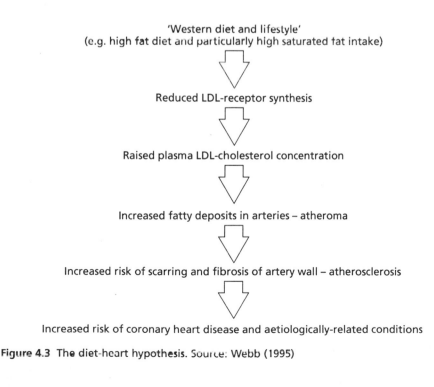

'Western diet and lifestyle'
(e.g. high fat diet and particularly high saturated fat intake)

Reduced LDL-receptor synthesis

Raised plasma LDL-cholesterol concentration

Increased fatty deposits in arteries – atheroma

Increased risk of scarring and fibrosis of artery wall – atherosclerosis

Increased risk of coronary heart disease and aetiologically-related conditions

Figure 4.3 The diet-heart hypothesis. Source: Webb (1995)

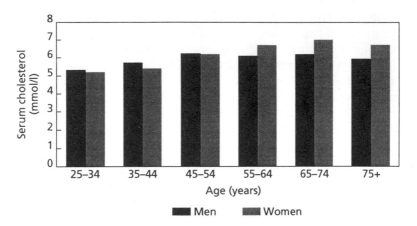

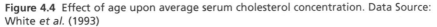

Figure 4.4 Effect of age upon average serum cholesterol concentration. Data Source: White *et al.* (1993)

EFFECTS OF AGEING UPON PLASMA CHOLESTEROL

Plasma total cholesterol tends to rise with age and this trend is most pronounced in postmenopausal women (see Figure 4.4). Prior to the menopause, average plasma cholesterol levels of women tend to be marginally lower than those of men but after the menopause the levels of women tend to be substantially higher than those of men. Table 4.5 shows the approximate distribution of serum cholesterol concentrations of those aged over 65 years in a sample of English adults. Only a fifth of English men and just 5% of women aged over 65 years have plasma cholesterol concentrations below 5.2 mmol/l; close to 40% of men and 60% of women over 65 years have levels above even the mildly elevated range, i.e. above 6.5 mmol/l. The role of diet in the treatment of elderly hyperlipidaemic patients is discussed in Chapter 8.

Table 4.5 Percentage distribution of English adults over 65 years according to their serum cholesterol concentration. Estimated from the data of White *et al.* (1993)

Serum cholesterol (mmol/l)	Men	Women
<5.2	19	5
>5.2 but <6.5	42	33
>6.5 but <7.8	36	38
7.8+	2	22

PLASMA CHOLESTEROL AND CORONARY HEART DISEASE – THE ROLE OF DIETARY FATS

Fatty acids are split up into three broad categories according to the number of double bonds that they contain: saturated – no double bonds; monounsaturated – one; and polyunsaturated – more than one double bond (reviewed in Webb, 1995). Table 4.6 shows the fatty acid composition of a number of different fats. Butter and lard, like most animal fat, are high in saturates and low in polyunsaturates; olive oil and canola oil are low in saturates and particularly high in monounsaturates; sunflower oil and soya oil are low in saturates and high in polyunsaturates.

According to the diet-heart hypothesis (Figure 4.3), high saturated fat intake is of prime importance in raising plasma cholesterol levels and so reduced consumption of saturated fat is the most effective dietary means of reducing it. There are potentially two ways of reducing saturated fat intake: either total fat intake can be reduced or there can be replacement of some saturated fat with unsaturated fat.

Reducing total fat intakes. Total fat consumption can be reduced by replacing some of the dietary fat with carbohydrate, reducing consumption of fatty meats, dairy products, margarine and cooking fats and increasing intake of cereals, potatoes and other vegetables and fruits. This approach is currently favoured in both UK and US nutrition education guidelines (e.g.

Table 4.6 Typical proportions (%) of saturated (S) monounsaturated (M) and polyunsaturated (P) fatty acids in different types of fat. Data source: Webb (1995)

Fat	%S	%M	%P	P:S ratio
Butter	64	33	3	0.05
Lard	47	44	9	0.2
Sunflower oil	14	34	53	4.0
Soyabean oil	15	26	59	4.0
Rapeseed* (canola)	7	60	33	5.0
Olive oil	15	73	13	0.8
Coconut oil	91**	7	2	0.02
Palm oil	48	44	8	0.2
Oil in salmon	28	42	30	1.0
Oil in mackerel	27	43	30	1.0

* low erucic acid variety
** includes large amount of short chain saturates

NRC, 1989a and COMA, 1991). Reduced fat consumption is seen as desirable on several grounds other than its effect on plasma cholesterol concentration. For example, it would tend to reduce the energy density of the diet and high fat diets have been associated with increased risk of some cancers such as bowel cancer. Increased consumption of cereals, vegetables and fruits is seen as desirable because it would, for example, increase intakes of dietary fibre, potassium and some antioxidants like vitamin C and β-carotene.

Substitution of unsaturated for saturated fat. In recent decades there have been substantial changes in the composition of dietary fats in the UK and USA. The ratio of polyunsaturated to saturated fatty acids in the UK diet has approximately doubled since the late 1970s largely because of substitution of soft margarine and vegetable oils for butter, hard margarine and animal-derived cooking fats (MAFF, 1993). Over 35 years ago, Keys *et al.* (1959) showed that switching from a diet high in saturated fat to one high in polyunsaturated fat was an effective means of reducing plasma cholesterol concentration. More recently, monounsaturated fats have been shown to have a similar cholesterol-lowering effect (e.g. Mattson and Grundy, 1985).

Several expert committees (e.g. NACNE, 1983; COMA, 1991; NRC, 1989) have voiced concerns about the long-term safety of diets very high in polyunsaturated fat and have suggested prudent upper limits to polyunsaturated fatty acid intakes that are close to the current levels of consumption in the USA and UK (6–7% of total calories). Even though older people may have lagged behind the general population in these changes in the composition of their dietary fats, further substantial increases in their polyunsaturated fat intake would seem to be undesirable. Concerns about the long-term safety of high monounsaturated fat intakes have not yet surfaced and so highly monounsaturated oils like olive oil and rapeseed (canola) oil currently have a very positive health image.

A number of other issues concerning the relationship between dietary fats, plasma cholesterol and coronary heart disease are listed below.

- Dietary cholesterol is now generally regarded as a relatively minor influence upon plasma cholesterol levels and UK guidelines contain no specific recommendations to lower dietary cholesterol intakes (e.g. COMA, 1991).
- Table 4.6 indicates that fish oil is high in polyunsaturates and low in saturates. Most of the polyunsaturates in fish oil have their first double bond between carbon 3 and carbon 4 (ω3 series) whereas most polyunsaturates in vegetable oils have their first double bond between carbons 6 and 7 (ω6 series). The ω3 fatty acids may have an anticoagulant effect, may reduce inflammation and may have favourable effects upon blood lipid levels (see Webb, 1995). There is convincing evidence that regular consumption of oily fish or fish oil supplements improves survival in those who have already experienced a myocardial infarction (Burr *et al.*, 1991).
- Some highly-publicised research has suggested that the trans fatty acids found in butter and most margarines may have a cholesterol-raising effect (Mensink and Katan, 1990) and that high consumption of these fatty acids may be associated with increased risk of coronary heart disease (Willett *et*

al., 1993). The largest proportion of trans fatty acids are found in the harder, cheaper margarines whose use has declined considerably in the UK in recent years.

CHOLESTEROL-LOWERING, SOME UNRESOLVED ISSUES

Many expert committees have considered the evidence and accepted the diet-heart hypothesis (e.g. COMA, 1991; NRC, 1989b). However, the high relative risk of CHD associated with any given level of elevated plasma cholesterol appears to decline with age (Shipley *et al.* 1991; Gordon and Rifkind, 1989). These observations strongly suggest that any potential benefit of a given lowering of plasma cholesterol declines as the age of the individual increases; older people may have less to gain from cholesterol-lowering than younger people. It has nevertheless been argued that as the general incidence of CHD rises with age, so a smaller reduction in relative risk in the elderly may actually amount to prevention of a larger absolute number of premature CHD deaths (COMA, 1992; Shipley *et al*, 1991). In other words, although any given individual elderly person may gain less than a younger person by cholesterol-lowering, because more elderly people die of CHD, the effect on total population mortality may still be higher in the elderly. Shipley *et al.* (1991) explained this apparent weakening of the predictive value of plasma cholesterol by suggesting that as risk factors like plasma cholesterol are predictors of premature death, then the less premature the death the less predictive the risk factor becomes.

The relationship between plasma cholesterol and total mortality is much less clear than that with CHD mortality. For example, in a 12-year cohort study of 15,000 middle-aged (45–64 years) Scottish men and women, Isles *et al.* (1989) found that total mortality was not related to plasma cholesterol concentration. A positive association between cholesterol values and CHD mortality was approximately balanced by an inverse relationship between cholesterol values and other causes of death, including cancer.

Jacobs *et al.* (1992) analysed the relationship between plasma cholesterol concentration and various causes of mortality in over 600,000 people. They found a U-curve of mortality associated with a rising plasma cholesterol concentration. At very low plasma concentrations (say <4 mmol/l) although death rate from CHD is very low, total mortality is raised due to increased death rate from non-cardiovascular causes like cancer. In young and middle-aged men there still appeared to be clear evidence of a net benefit from a lowering of average cholesterol concentration. Nevertheless, these results raise doubts about whether cholesterol-lowering is holistically beneficial for all subgroups of the population. In women, for example, there was an essentially flat relationship between total mortality and plasma cholesterol concentration. In women, even cardiovascular mortality was not significantly associated with cholesterol level; as cholesterol concentration fell so CHD mortality also fell but this was counterbalanced by a rise in mortality from stroke. Hulley *et al.* (1992), in an editorial discussion of these results, suggested that it might be time to consider whether universal cholesterol-lowering advice could still be ethically justified. They particularly questioned the value of cholesterol-lowering in women (a substantial majority of the over 65s).

Cholesterol-lowering trials have frequently produced reductions in the number of coronary incidents in the intervention group but any decline in CHD mortality is generally not statistically significant and there is in general no effect on total mortality. A non-significant decline in mortality from CHD is often roughly balanced by a non significant increase in deaths from other causes (Dunnigan, 1993).

Smith et al. (1993) combined the results of 35 controlled trials of cholesterol-lowering interventions (three-quarters of which involved the use of cholesterol-lowering drugs). They concluded that net benefit in terms of reduced all-cause mortality was confined to those trials where the death rate from CHD was extremely high so only those at very high risk of CHD had been shown to gain net benefit from individual, cholesterol-lowering intervention. Some of those at low initial risk may suffer net harm from intervention, especially if cholesterol-lowering drugs are used. This point needs to be carefully considered before active intervention (especially the use of cholesterol-lowering drugs) is contemplated in elderly women, almost a quarter of whom have plasma cholesterol concentrations within the hypercholesteraemic range (see Chapter 8 for further discussion).

One of the arguments used most frequently to explain the inability to demonstrate holistic benefit in cholesterol-lowering trials, is that it is not possible to use a large enough sample for long enough to get a statistically significant reduction in total mortality. This is another way of saying that the risk of dying during the duration of the trial is only minutely affected by the intervention. The decline in the predictive value of high plasma cholesterol even for CHD in the elderly might suggest that individual elderly people have even less to gain from cholesterol-lowering.

The lack of success in some cholesterol-lowering intervention trials has been explained by suggesting that intervention was started too late, i.e. the subjects were too old to gain significant benefit from the intervention. This again implies that the benefits of cholesterol-lowering are likely to be greatest in younger people and, in the light of the earlier discussion, particularly in younger men.

CONCLUSIONS

In the longer term, health promotion may reduce the average plasma cholesterol of the adult population and reduce the tendency of cholesterol levels to rise with age. This reduction in cholesterol levels would be expected to reduce mortality and morbidity from coronary heart disease and, particularly amongst men, might be expected to increase longevity and increase expectation of life without disability.

Most elderly people have serum cholesterol levels that are considered to be higher than ideal. There is, however, no compelling evidence that any other than a small minority at very high risk of myocardial infarction (e.g. those with existing CHD or severe hyperlipidaemia and family history of premature

CHD) will gain significant holistic benefit from individual, specifically cho-lesterol-lowering, interventions. This means that the case for general screening of plasma cholesterol levels in elderly people is not a substantial one. Only about 2% of elderly men are hypercholesteraemic (Table 4.5) and although the figure is much higher in elderly women the relationship between cholesterol level and mortality in women is much less clear and much less studied than that in men. Cholesterol screening is expensive and may well cause considerable anxiety to the majority of elderly people if they are told that their cholesterol level is elevated. The financial costs of treatment and the deleterious effects on the quality of life of elderly people may be considerable. If treatment involves the use of drugs the possible risks of drug therapy have to be considered.

The uncertainties discussed above did not convince the COMA (1992) expert working party that the elderly population should be excluded from the cholesterol-lowering recommendations directed at the general adult popula-tion. One of the recommendations of this group was that 'elderly people should be encouraged to adopt diets which moderate their plasma cholesterol levels'. It is argued that even though the individual risk reduction may be smaller in the elderly, at the population level the potential reduction in the number of CHD deaths may be greater. It must be said, however, that as with many other aspects of nutrition in the elderly, the evidence upon which this recommendation is based is very limited.

Table 4.7 shows a number of measures that might be expected to contribute to a lowering of plasma cholesterol and/or coronary heart disease. Most of these measures are suggested for other reasons elsewhere in this chapter; they

Table 4.7 Some dietary and related measures that have been suggested by expert commit-tees that may lower plasma cholesterol concentration and/or reduce the risk of coronary heart disease

Increase energy expenditure by increased physical activity
Maintain an 'ideal' body weight
Reduce fat consumption to 35% or even 30% of total calories and replace existing fat above this level with starch foods
Reduce saturated fat intake to 15% or even 10% of total calories
Reduce dietary salt consumption (in order to reduce the prevalence of hypertension)
Moderate excessive alcohol consumption
Increase consumption of fruits and vegetables (thus increasing consumption of soluble fibre, antioxidant vitamins and potassium)
Regular consumption of fatty fish
Reduced cigarette smoking

can thus be justified irrespective of the benefits or otherwise of cholesterol-lowering in elderly adults. Implementation of these measures should together lead to a reduction in cholesterol levels and the age-specific incidence of CHD in the elderly. When taken together they should increase longevity and increase the expectation of life without disability.

If we focus particularly upon dietary fats, it has already been suggested that there are many grounds for advising elderly people to take less of their calories as fat and more as complex carbohydrate irrespective of its effects upon plasma cholesterol. For example, it might be expected to:

- improve glucose tolerance
- increase intakes of dietary fibre and thus improve bowel function
- contribute to a reduction in levels of overweight and obesity in the elderly.

Should elderly people be encouraged to alter the composition of their dietary fats? Increases in the consumption of ω6 polyunsaturates above the current consumption levels of the rest of the adult population would seem to be undesirable. Although monunsaturated fatty acids are currently viewed more favourably there is no guarantee that, in years to come, concerns about the safety of diets very high in monounsaturates will not surface. One of the traditional characteristics of a good diet has been diversity. Eating a wide variety of foods increases the probability that the requirements for all of the essential nutrients will be met and reduces the probability that any potentially toxic components in individual foods will be consumed in hazardous amounts. Perhaps the low-risk option is for elderly people and those catering for the elderly to apply this general principle of diversity to dietary fats. This would involve mixing fats from different sources so that no one type of fatty acid becomes too dominant in the diet.

For those elderly people who like oily fish, regular inclusion of oily fish in the diet (one or two portions per week) may offer potential benefits at low risk. COMA (1992) specifically recommended that elderly people should be encouraged to consume oily fish to reduce their risk of thrombosis. On the basis of current evidence, concentrated fish oil supplements are probably best reserved for those identified at high and immediate risk of myocardial infarction or those with some types of hyperlipidaemia (see Chapter 8). A short review of fish oils may be found in Webb (1995).

For most elderly people, the specific restriction of cholesterol-rich foods would seem undesirable as these are often particularly rich in essential nutrients, e.g. eggs, liver, milk, cheese and some shellfish are all relatively high in cholesterol but are excellent sources of certain essential nutrients. Dietary adequacy assumes a much higher priority in older people than it does for younger adults.

Alcohol consumption

In Chapter 1, data drawn from *Family Spending 1992* and from the *National Food Survey* (MAFF, 1993) indicated that elderly people spent less upon alcohol than younger adults, both in absolute terms, and as a proportion of total spending. Thus in 1992, per capita expenditure upon alcoholic drinks in old age pensioner households (OAP) was only 40–45% of that in all one- and two-adult households. Alcohol represented only about 4% of total food and drink expenditure in OAP households but double this proportion in the comparison groups (see Table 1.10).

In the case of alcohol, individual consumption is considered to be more important than population averages (NACNE, 1983). It has been a fairly consistent finding in epidemiological studies that low to moderate alcohol consumption is associated with reduced total and heart disease mortality as compared to complete abstinence. On the other hand, high alcohol consumption is associated with steep increases in total mortality due to increases in cancer, liver disease, accidents and strokes. The health promotion objective with alcohol is, therefore, to try to truncate the distribution of alcohol intakes that is to reduce the intake of high consumers rather than to shift the whole distribution of alcohol intakes downwards as is the aim in several other areas of nutrition education (fat and salt consumption).

At the present time, 21 units of alcohol per week is widely regarded as a safe level of consumption for men and 14 units per week for women. A unit of alcohol is a half pint of ordinary beer, a small glass of wine or a single measure of spirits. If alcohol consumption is spread reasonably evenly throughout the week then levels up to 60% higher than these maxima may be regarded as acceptable and pose little direct threat to the health of older adults. Table 4.8 indicates the distribution of elderly English adults amongst different alcohol consumption categories. In general, this suggests that alcohol consumption in excess of current guidelines is less prevalent amongst older adults than amongst the younger adult population. Nevertheless, around 20% of elderly men drink in excess of the current recommended maximum and nearly 10% drink in excess of 35 units per week. The data in Table 4.8 suggests that excessive drinking amongst elderly women is relatively uncommon.

A 10–12 year Danish cohort study (Gronbaek et al., 1994) confirmed the U-shaped relationship between total mortality and alcohol consumption, with lowest relative mortality risk in those consuming 1–6 units of alcohol per week. This study also reported that only with weekly alcohol consumption in excess of 42 units per week was total mortality significantly higher than in those consuming low amounts of alcohol. This study found that age did not change the relationship between mortality risk and alcohol consumption. Some other studies in the USA (e.g. Klatsky et al., 1992) have reported that the relative risk of dying as a result of alcohol consumption is higher in younger people than older people because of the alcohol-related increase in deaths from violence and traffic accidents in younger adults. Gronbaek et al. (1994) suggest that this difference in findings between the American and Danish studies may be because accidents and violence are less prominent as causes of death amongst young Danes than amongst young Americans.

Despite the apparent benefits of low or even moderate alcohol consumption, health promotion guidelines do not usually go so far as to recommend

Table 4.8 Distribution of elderly people in England between different alcohol consumption categories, comparison with the adult population in general. All values are a percentage of the people in the category. Data source: White *et al.* (1993)

| | Consumption category | | | |
	Nil	low/moderate	fairly high	high
Men				
All 16+ years	17	55	14	14
65-74 years	25	55	11	9
75+ years	37	47	10	7
Women				
All 16+ years	35	53	8	5
65-74 years	50	46	4	–
75+ years	55	38	3	–

Key

Nil = < 1 unit per week
Low/moderate = 1–21♂; 1–14♀
Fairly high = 22–35♂; 15–25♀
High = 35+♂; 25+♀

regular alcohol consumption by current abstainers. The social and medical dangers of excess alcohol consumption are very clear and severe and many people lack the ability to regulate their consumption once they start to drink regularly. Bored or lonely elderly people who drink regularly might well be particularly prone to excessive use. One other important point to bear in mind is that alcoholic drinks contribute calories to the diet but few nutrients. They thus tend to lower the nutrient density of the diet. This may be an important additional problem in those elderly people whose energy requirements are low, making it difficult for them to satisfy their needs for other essential nutrients. Many nutrient deficiencies that are otherwise rare in industrial countries are regularly found in alcoholics. Current UK taxation policy also makes alcohol a relatively expensive commodity and so in elderly people with very restricted incomes, alcohol can be a severe drain on their limited financial resources, leaving even less money to spend on food and other essentials. The problem of alcohol misuse and its management in the elderly is briefly reviewed by Dunn (1994).

The UK safe drinking recommendations have now been increased by 7 units per week for both men and women (♂ now 28, ♀ now 21). This new Department of Health statement also contains positive encouragement for older people who don't drink to consider taking a regular drink (one or two units per day).

Cigarette smoking

A detailed discussion of cigarette smoking and its effects upon health is clearly inappropriate in a nutrition text. Nevertheless, given its importance as a risk factor for heart disease, cancer and strokes, some brief review of the smoking habits of the elderly is necessary for the completeness of this review of risk factors in the elderly. It is also clear that risk factors should not be considered in isolation because they tend to interact. Combinations of elevated risk factors produce increases in total risk that may be far higher than the sum of each of the individual increases in risk. Thus, for example, a high fat diet may be more significant for smokers than non-smokers.

Table 4.9 The prevalence of cigarette smoking in various age categories of English adults. Data source: White *et al.* (1993)

	Age (years)				
Smoking category	16–24	35–44	55–64	65–74	75+
Men (%)					
Smokers	34	32	30	27	14
Ex-smokers	5	26	49	55	60
Non-smokers	61	42	21	18	26
Women (%)					
Smokers	35	30	24	17	15
Ex-smokers	5	20	24	39	26
Non-smokers	61	50	52	44	59

Older people spend less upon tobacco than younger adults (see Table 1.10). Table 4.9 shows the proportion of various age groups of English adults who are currently regular smokers or ex-smokers. In general, the prevalence of smoking declines with age. However, given the past high prevalence of this habit in the UK the proportion of ex-smokers tends to rise with age. One factor in the apparent decline in the popularity of smoking with age is the much higher death rates of smokers in the younger age groups so that fewer smokers survive into old age.

A summary of current nutrition education guidelines – are they suitable for older adults?

Table 4.10 shows the 'ideal' diet as suggested by the long term nutrition education targets of the National Advisory Committee on Nutrition Education (NACNE, 1983) and compares it to the actual diet of British adults as measured by weighed inventory (Gregory *et al.*, 1990). This ideal diet would also be consistent with nutrition education guidelines suggested in the USA (e.g. NRC, 1989a) and other industrialised countries. The major changes necessary to meet these targets are a substantial reduction in the proportion of total energy that is derived from fat, saturated fat and sugars with a commensurate increase in the proportion derived from starches. Substantial reductions in average salt intake, a substantial increase in fibre intake and moderation of alcohol intake are also recommended.

The figures for the current diet in Table 4.10 are for adults below 65 years and no recent, comparable figures are available for older adults in the UK. Whether they represent a reasonable estimate of the diet composition of older adults is not easy to judge. The last consumption survey of older UK adults was in 1967–1968 (DHSS, 1972), and the general conclusion was that the diets of older people were basically similar to those of other adults. In order to effect the compositional changes necessary to meet the 'ideal' values in Table 4.10 consumption of fats, sweets, meat and dairy foods must decline whilst those of cereals, fruits and vegetable must increase. Evidence presented in Chapter 1 suggested that, if anything, the diets of older adults might be slightly further from the target values than those of younger adults. OAP households spend much less upon fruits and vegetables and more on fats and sugar than other adult households.

Table 4.10 Current estimates of the average UK adult (16–64 years) diet composition compared with the 'ideal' of NACNE (1983). Values are % of total energy unless otherwise stated. Data source: Webb (1995)

Nutrient	Current	Ideal
Fat	38	30
Saturated fat	16	10
Protein	14	11
Total carbohydrate	42	55
Sugars	18	10
Alcohol	6	4
Salt (g/day)	9	6
Fibre (g/day)*	20	30

*Precise numerical values for fibre depend upon definition and method of estimation; using current estimations of non-starch polysaccharide, current and ideal values of 12 g and 18 g/day could be substituted.

Table 4.11 shows a selective comparison of the nutrient composition of the household food purchases of old age pensioner (OAP) and one- and two-adult households. The absolute numerical values in Tables 4.10 and 4.11 are not directly comparable because the *National Food Survey* used to construct Table 4.11 measures the composition of household food purchases whereas the dietary survey used to construct Table 4.10 used a weighed inventory of food as consumed. What Table 4.11 can indicate is any gross difference in the composition of food purchased by older adults compared to adults as a whole and thus likely differences in the consumption of young and old adults. In fact Table 4.11 shows a striking similarity between the composition of the food consumed by the three types of household. The only difference of note is the relatively high consumption of non-milk extrinsic sugars in the OAPs. Even this difference narrows when one includes the higher contribution of sugars from drinks and confectionary in the one- and two-adult households. There is also slightly lower consumption by the older groups of those antioxidant nutrients listed in the NFS; in the case of β-carotene, the difference is large.

Table 4.11 A comparison of the daily nutritional content of household food purchases of old age pensioner households (OAP) and all one or two adult only households. Data source: MAFF (1993)

	Household type		
Nutrient	1 adult	2 adult	OAP
Energy (kcal)	2110	2110	2170
Protein (g)	71	72	70
(% energy)	13.5	13.8	12.9
Fat (g)	97	98	100
(% energy)	41.3	41.7	41.5
Saturated fat (g)	39	39	41
(% energy)	16.6	16.5	16.8
P:S ratio	0.39	0.41	0.38
Carbohydrate (g)	254	250	263
(% energy)	45.2	44.5	45.6
Non milk extrinsic sugars (g)	67	65	77
(% energy)	11.9	11.6	13.3
Salt (g)	7.3	7.2	6.9
Selected antioxidant nutrients			
Zinc (mg)	9.0	9.1	8.7
Vitamin C (mg)	55	61	52
β-carotene (mg)	2020	2100	1780

This is a reflection of the reduced consumption of coloured vegetables and fruits in the OAP households. The limitations of the *National Food Survey* as a measure of food consumption were discussed in Chapter 1 and these problems underline the need for a comprehensive survey of the dietary practices of older people.

The dietary changes suggested by Table 4.10 would be expected to produce a variety of health benefits, including those listed below.

- **Reduced levels of overweight** and obesity because of the reduced energy density or increased bulkiness of the diet.
- **Reduced average blood pressure** and reduced incidence of hypertension because of reductions in overweight, reduced salt intake, moderation of alcohol intakes and possibly increased potassium intakes.
- **Reduced incidence of CHD** because of the resultant moderation of plasma cholesterol and the reductions in overweight and hypertension.
- **Reduced cancer incidence**, as a result of several of these measures, such as: reduced fat intake and/or increased fibre (bowel cancer?), reduced salt intake (gastric cancer?), moderation of alcohol intake (cancers of the mouth, throat, liver and bowel); increased consumption of fruits and vegetables may have a general protective effect perhaps because of the antioxidant vitamins that they provide.
- **Improved bowel function** because of the increased intake of dietary fibre leading to a decrease in several bowel disorders such as constipation, diverticulosis and haemorrhoids (piles).
- **Improved glucose tolerance** and reduced prevalence of diabetes because of the reductions in body weight, the increased proportion of dietary energy derived from carbohydrate and the increased intake of dietary fibre.
- **Reduced prevalence of dental caries** because of the reduced sugar intakes.

Many of these expected benefits would appear from earlier discussions in this chapter and in Chapter 3 to be particularly advantageous for older people, such as the improvements in glucose tolerance, the reduction in blood pressure and hypertension and the improvements in bowel function. None of them are irrelevant to the elderly; even the effects on dental caries are becoming more relevant as more people are retaining their own teeth into old age. Thus it would seem that, in general qualitative terms, the direction of change suggested by these guidelines is equally appropriate to the 'young elderly' and those in relatively good health. COMA (1992) specifically listed the fibre, salt and sugar recommendations as being appropriate for the elderly and they also recommended a diet that would moderate plasma cholesterol levels.

It is also clear, however, that some of the quantitative recommendations listed in Table 4.10 are probably unrealistic for the population as a whole. They are achievable by individuals who are highly motivated and knowledgeable about food and nutrition but they are unlikely to be more widely achieved. Almost no British adults meet the recommendations for fat and saturated fat in Table 4.10 (Gregory *et al.*, 1990). Other UK expert groups (COMA, 1984 and 1991) have suggested a figure of 35% of food energy from fat as a more realistic target than the 30% figure given in Table 4.10. Even this more modest figure was suggested as a goal for the year 2005 in *The health of the nation* (DH, 1992). To implement both the sugar and fat recommendations in Table 4.10 would involve more than doubling the proportion of energy from starch. This would greatly increase the bulk of the diet and probably reduce its palatability to most people. In practice, in free-living and affluent populations, there tends to be an inverse relationship between fat and sugar consumption, the so called 'sugar-fat seesaw' (McColl, 1988). This might tend to make the sugar and fat recommendations almost mutually exclusive. With younger adults, and particularly younger men, the fat recommendations are generally seen as the nutrition education priority.

How realistic and appropriate are the quantitative targets in Table 4.10 for elderly people?

- There is a general tendency for older people to lag behind the general population trends in dietary change. Recommendations that are ambitious or unrealistic in general are probably even more so in the elderly. Attempts to induce very large changes in the diets of elderly people are likely to have more effects upon their cultural security than in the young. Reductions in the pleasure gained from food and drink may have a disproportionate impact on the total quality of life in those elderly people whose other pleasures have been reduced by infirmity or isolation.
- The fat and sugar recommendations may be difficult to implement together. Should fat be the nutrition education priority in older people, as it is in younger adults? There is little evidence upon which to base a reasoned answer to this question.
- Can elderly people afford to make the changes suggested by Table 4.10? The relative poverty of many elderly people was seen in Chapter 1. Some changes towards 'healthier eating' require little or no increased expenditure (e.g. use of oil rather than lard for cooking) but money is a major barrier towards further changes towards a low-fat, high fibre diet in poorer groups. Fatty and sugary foods are more cost-effective suppliers of dietary energy than fruits and fresh vegetables (Leather, 1992). If high fat, high sugar foods are replaced by starchy staples, in theory a healthy diet could be cheaper than the current diet. However, if as is more likely, people try to choose a healthier diet whilst staying close to current cultural eating patterns (by buying leaner meat, wholemeal bread, more fruit and fresh vegetables) then this is will substantially increase food costs (Groom, 1993). These increases in the cost of a healthier diet are beyond the economic means of many elderly people.
- There may be a substantial minority of elderly people for whom even the general qualitative shifts suggested in Table 4.10 may be inappropriate, or at least low priority – the very elderly, the frail, those whose appetite is poor, those who are underweight or losing weight, the sick elderly. The overriding priority in these people is to maintain or increase the flow of energy and essential nutrients. Measures which increase dietary bulk and reduce its palatability are likely to exacerbate these problems. The consumption of nutrient-rich foods like eggs, milk and meat needs to be

encouraged whatever the predicted effect upon plasma cholesterol. Of course, some measures like reduced sugar consumption to increase the nutrient density of the diet and increased fibre consumption may still be theoretically desirable even in this group. However, the practical result of such changes may be to further reduce food intake and accelerate weight loss. Ensuring that food is familiar, acceptable, tasty and rich in energy and nutrients outweighs any healthy eating considerations; this principle applies to sick and injured people generally (KFC, 1992).

The nutritional status of the elderly population

Aims and scope of the chapter

This chapter reviews current information on the nutritional status of elderly people in affluent countries, like the UK and USA. Current estimates of the nutritional needs of elderly people are summarised and there is discussion of how fully these estimated needs are being met by current intakes. The social and medical factors that predispose certain elderly people to malnutrition are also considered. This review includes a discussion of the nutritional status of elderly hospital patients and the effects that drugs may have upon nutritional status. The aims of the chapter are:

- to review current estimates of the nutritional needs of elderly people and how these are thought to differ from those of younger adults
- to quantify both the prevalence of undernutrition in elderly populations within affluent countries and to identify those nutrients that are most likely to be consumed in inadequate or marginal amounts
- to highlight some of the shortcomings in our current knowledge of the nutritional needs and status of elderly people; this should help to identify some of the priority topics for future research
- to highlight the social, medical, and nutritional factors that contribute to a relatively high prevalence of malnutrition in the elderly and thus to facilitate recognition of those elderly people most at risk of undernutrition
- to identify some population strategies that could improve the nutritional status of elderly people

- to review the prevalence and causes of malnutrition amongst elderly hospital patients
- to review the interactions between diet and drugs and the effects drugs may have upon the nutritional status of elderly people.

Estimating nutrient needs – Dietary Reference Values

General overview

An essential prerequisite for judging the nutritional status of any population or group is some standard yardstick of adequacy against which measured intakes or nutrient supplies can be compared. Many governments and other agencies publish sets of dietary standards which are intended to be used as such a yardstick. These standards are set by panels of national or international nutrition experts who attempt to estimate the requirements of each age and sex subgroup of the population for each of the essential nutrients. In the UK these standards are called Dietary Reference Values, DRVs (COMA, 1991) and in the US they are still known by the traditional name of Recommended Dietary Allowances, RDAs (NRC, 1989a).

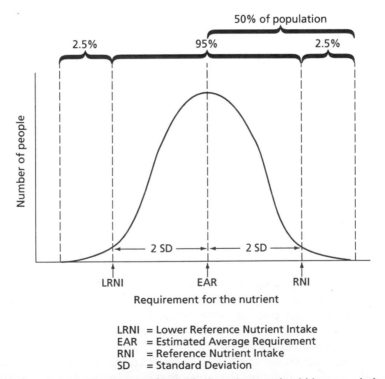

LRNI = Lower Reference Nutrient Intake
EAR = Estimated Average Requirement
RNI = Reference Nutrient Intake
SD   = Standard Deviation

Figure 5.1 A 'normal' distribution of individual nutrient needs within a population with the theoretical positions of the UK Dietary Reference Values. Source: Webb (1994)

In the UK system, three values are given for most essential nutrients, and there are around 30 population subgroups. The assumption is that, within any given population group, the requirement for most nutrients is distributed 'normally' (in the statistical sense) around a mean or average requirement (see Figure 5.1). The standard deviation is a precisely defined statistical measure of the variation around a mean or average value and, in a 'normal' distribution, 95% of values should lie within a range of two standard deviations on either side of the mean or average value. The three Dietary Reference Values given for most essential nutrients in the UK are:

- **Estimated Average Requirement (EAR)**
  The panel's estimate of **average need** for the nutrient within the particular population subgroup.
- **Reference Nutrient Intake (RNI)**
  A value that is estimated to be **two standard deviations above the EAR** – this value should theoretically be sufficient to meet the needs of 97.5% of the group.
- **Lower Reference Nutrient Intake (LRNI)**
  A value estimated to be **two standard deviations below the EAR** – this amount should theoretically be sufficient to meet the needs of only 2.5% of the population group.

The RNI is the most widely used of these three values because it is essentially equivalent to the traditional RDA (Recommended Dietary Allowance) that is still used in other countries, like the USA. Both the RDA and RNI represent the estimated needs of those people with a particularly high need for the nutrient. If a healthy person is consuming more than the RNI/RDA for any nutrient then it is assumed they are receiving adequate amounts of that nutrient. This is a relatively safe assumption, even though theoretically 2.5% of the population should require more than the RNI/RDA; these values tend to be estimated generously with a strong tendency to err on the high side.

The other two values in the new British system (first introduced in COMA, 1991) are intended to assist in the interpretation of measured intakes that are below the RNI. If an individual is consuming the LRNI or less, then their intake of that nutrient is considered to be almost certainly inadequate. If they are consuming their EAR, then there is a roughly 50% chance that they are meeting their individual needs according to the criterion of need used by the DRV panel. When a measured intake falls between the LRNI and the RNI it is possible to make a precise estimate of the probability that this person is receiving an adequate supply of that nutrient.

In the case of energy, the RDA has traditionally been set at the best estimate of average requirement rather than, as with most nutrients, the estimated requirement of those with the highest needs. This practice has been followed in the latest edition of the American RDAs (NRC, 1989a). Consistent with this practice, the UK panel (COMA, 1991) gives only an EAR for energy and not an RNI. The rationale for only using average values, when dealing with estimated energy requirements, is that setting high 'target' values, (like an RNI/RDA based upon estimates of highest requirements) might encourage overconsumption and thus obesity. It might also lead to wasteful overprovision, if they were used to estimate the food requirements of a group. It is assumed that in healthy people, physiological hunger mechanisms will ensure that people will generally consume sufficient energy to meet their needs, provided that food is available and that these mechanisms are not wilfully overridden (as in dieting). This assumption may be less secure in elderly people than in younger adults. Poor appetite, weight loss and underweight are common problems in the elderly and particularly in the frail and very elderly. The acuity of the hunger mechanism, in common with thirst and some other homeostatic mechanisms, may decline with age.

For some nutrients, where information about requirements is deemed insufficient to set reliable RDAs or DRVs, then both the UK and USA panels use the term 'safe intake': an intake, or often a range of intakes, that should be sufficient to prevent deficiency without risk of toxicity.

Unlike the previous editions, the current UK DRVs include reference values for fat and carbohydrate. These are in the form of desirable population average intakes for:

• total fat
• saturated, monounsaturated and polyunsaturated fatty acids
• total carbohydrate
• added sugars
• starch and intrinsic sugars
• non-starch polysaccharide or fibre.

Minimum and maximum target values for individuals are also set for the polyunsaturated fatty acids and non-starch polysaccharide. These values break new ground for the dietary standards in that their purpose is not the traditional one of setting standards of adequacy. They are primarily aimed at reducing mortality and morbidity from the degenerative 'diseases of industrialisation', e.g. heart disease, maturity onset diabetes and cancer. The appropriateness of many of these values for older people was discussed in Chapter 4.

Limitations of dietary standards

Webb (1994 and 1995) has reviewed dietary standards and gives extended discussion of the errors and uncertainties involved in setting them. Despite the apparently precise statistical definitions given above, these reference values cannot be precisely and objectively measured, they are dependent to a great extent upon the scientific judgement of the members of expert committees. Not surprisingly, therefore, the values may vary widely from country to country and they may fluctuate over time. For example, in the USA the RDA for vitamin C for an adult male is 50% higher than the corresponding RNI in the UK; the RDA for calcium in a 20-year-old woman is over 70% higher than the corresponding UK RNI. Tables 5.1 and 5.2 give further examples of differences between USA and UK dietary standards that relate specifically to older people.

Table 5.1 UK and US Dietary Reference Values for energy in older adults. Data sources: COMA (1991); NRC (1989a)

Age (years)	Men kcal (MJ)	Women kcal (MJ)
	United Kingdom (EAR)	
19–50	2550 (10.60)	1940 (8.10)
51–59	2550 (10.60)	1900 (8.00)
60–64	2380 (9.93)	1900 (7.99)
65–74	2330 (9.71)	1900 (7.96)
75+	2100 (8.77)	1810 (7.61)
	United States (RDA)	
25–50	2900 (12.12)	2200 (9.20)
51+	2300 (9.61)	1900 (7.94)

One obvious area of uncertainty is in the choice of criteria used to define adequacy. The minimum criterion for many nutrients could be the amount necessary to prevent overt symptoms of any deficiency disease and this can often be measured with some precision. However, like the committees in many other countries, the UK panel on DRVs clearly felt that an affluent society should expect more than the basic avoidance of overt deficiency diseases. The UK panel set its values to allow for a degree of storage of the nutrient so that periods of low intake or increased requirement could be tolerated without immediate detriment to health. DRVs are intended to be used with healthy people and no allowance is made for the effects of illness or drug therapy upon nutrient needs. Many elderly people have some chronic condition and/or take regular medication; the effects upon nutrient needs are often unquantified and rarely considered.

Such a necessarily vague definition of adequacy as that given above clearly creates considerable scope for variation in estimating the need for any given nutrient. In addition, there are also errors and uncertainties in the methods used to measure the intake required to fulfil any defined criterion of adequacy and in estimating the standard deviation of requirement. These uncertainties need to be borne in mind when using DRVs. There is a particular need to be cautious when using DRVs to assess the nutritional status or needs of individuals rather than groups.

The panels that set DRVs will be conscious that if they set values below the true level of adequacy this will render them completely useless for their intended purposes. This means that there will be a strong temptation to err on the high side, because a moderate excess of most nutrients is not directly harmful. It should also be borne in mind that the underlying criterion used in

Table 5.2 A comparison of UK RNIs and US RDAs for selected nutrients for elderly adults. Values in parentheses are the US values as a percentage of the UK values. Data sources: COMA (1991) and NRC (1989a)

	Male		Female	
	UK	US	UK	US
Protein (g)	53.3	63 (118)	46.5	50 (108)
Vitamin A (µg)	700	1000 (143)	600	800 (133)
Vitamin D (µg)	10*	5 (50)	10*	5 (50)
Vitamin C (mg)	40	60 (150)	40	60 (150)
Thiamin (mg)	0.9	1.2 (133)	0.8	1.0 (125)
Riboflavin (mg)	1.3	1.4 (108)	1.1	1.2 (109)
Niacin (mg)	16	15 (94)	12	13 (108)
Folate (µg)	200	200 (100)	200	200 (100)
Vitamin B_{12} (µg)	1.5	2 (133)	1.5	2 (133)
Calcium (mg)	700	800 (114)	700	800 (114)
Iron (mg)	8.7	10 (115)	8.7	10 (115)
Zinc (mg)	9.5	15 (158)	7.0	12 (171)

* over 65 years only, no RNI for younger adults

setting these standards remains prevention of deficiency rather than optimising health. The additional criterion of ensuring adequate storage of nutrients represents a margin of safety compared to simple disease prevention. As a general rule, however, the UK panel did not take into account claims of beneficial effects of very high intakes of particular nutrients, of issues like:

- the possible effect of large doses of vitamin C in maximising resistance to infection
- the suggestion that very high intakes of vitamin E may reduce the risk of heart disease
- the suggestion that large calcium supplements may increase bone density and reduce the risk of osteoporosis.

Many of the general uncertainties involved in setting dietary standards are even greater when dealing with the needs of the elderly. There have been comparatively few studies that have attempted to directly assess the nutrient needs of elderly people. Are the indices of satisfactory nutrient status used in younger adults still valid in the elderly and very elderly? The COMA (1992) report on the nutrition of the elderly recommended that there needed to be more research aimed at quantifying:

- the energy requirements of elderly people and particularly those who are thin
- the effects of health status on the energy requirements of elderly people
- the protein requirements of elderly people
- the micronutrient requirements of elderly people.

DRVs for elderly people

How are energy needs estimated?

The energy requirements of population groups are usually estimated by first calculating the expected average basal metabolic rate (BMR) and then multiplying this by some factor to allow for the physical activity level (PAL) of the group. The BMR is the energy expenditure at rest, under certain specified conditions, and it represents the energy required to maintain the essential body functions like breathing and blood circulation. It is usually estimated by using an equation that predicts metabolic rate from either body weight alone or from body weight in conjunction with one or more extra parameters (e.g. height and age). The equations of Schofield *et al.* (1985) are well known and are now widely used for this purpose, although they are not considered reliable enough for predictive purposes in elderly subjects (COMA, 1991). As illustrative examples, the equations used by COMA (1991) to predict the BMRs of men and women aged over 75 years are shown below.

$$\male \, BMR = (0.0350) \times W + 3.434$$
$$\female \, BMR = (0.0410) \times W + 2.610$$

Where: W = body weight (kg)
and BMR = basal metabolic rate (MJ/day)

COMA (1991) and NRC (1989a) both chose a rather arbitrary multiple of 1.5 times the BMR to allow for physical activity (PAL) and thus to predict the average total energy requirement of elderly people. There is some discussion of the rationale for the use of this PAL multiple later in the chapter.

Effects of age upon BMR and activity level

Both physical activity levels and the BMR tend to decline with age and consequently energy requirements also tend to decline with age. Figure 5.2 shows the estimated decline in BMR with age in British adults. This fall in BMR probably reflects a decline in the amount of lean tissue because when BMR is expressed per kilogram of fat-free mass, this decline in BMR with age is not apparent (COMA, 1992). The decline in body oxygen consumption with age almost exactly reflects the decline in the cellular mass (Kenney, 1989). If one compares the typical body composition of a young person with an elderly one, then solid cellular material (lean tissue) declines as a proportion of the

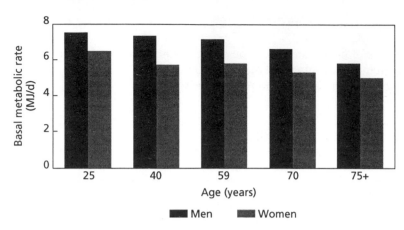

Figure 5.2 Changes in BMR with age. Data source: COMA (1992).

total body weight whereas metabolically inert fat makes up a higher proportion of the body weight (see Chapter 3). This decline in fat-free mass with age may itself be largely a consequence of the decline in physical activity with age (COMA, 1992).

There is ample evidence that over the last 30–40 years there has been a considerable decline in the general activity of the whole UK population. The *National Food Survey* shows that the energy value of household food purchases declined from around 2600 kcal per person per day in the early 1960s to only about 1850 kcal per day in the early 1990s. Even though the NFS is an imperfect measure of total food intake, a change of this magnitude indicates very significant decreases in energy consumption and when coupled with increasing levels of overweight and obesity points to very substantial decreases in energy expenditure. In common with the rest of the population, the elderly are also less active now than in previous decades (COMA, 1992). Lack of good data about past activity levels, energy expenditure, or even the energy intakes of large representative samples of elderly people, makes quantification of this decline difficult. The steep decline in average activity level with age has been discussed in Chapter 4.

Current energy EARs/RDAs for elderly adults

Table 5.1 shows the current UK EARs for energy in older adults and the corresponding American RDAs. In setting the UK values, COMA (1991) acknowledged that activity level was a major determinant of energy requirement. COMA was, however, concerned that if it was seen to recommend intakes of energy that truly reflected the very low expenditure of many inactive elderly people, then total food intake would be so low as to make inadequacy of some essential nutrients probable. COMA did not, therefore, use a declining multiple (i.e. the PAL) of BMR with age; for people over 60 years it used a figure of 1.5 times the calculated BMR to arrive at the EAR. For people under 60 years it used a multiple of only 1.4 times the BMR. This

Table 5.3 Differences between Dietary Reference Values for elderly adults (over 50 years) and those of younger adults. For those nutrients not listed here, the values for younger and older adults are the same

Nutrient	RNIs – United Kingdom			
	Male		Female	
	19–50 years	50+	19–50 years	50+
Protein (g)	55.5	53.3	45.0	46.5
Thiamin (mg)	1.0	0.9	–	–
Niacin (mg)	17.0	16.0	13.0	12.0
Vitamin D* (µg)	0	10.0	0	10.0
Iron (mg)	–	–	14.8	8.7
	RDAs – United States			
Thiamin(mg)	1.5	1.2	1.1	1.0
Riboflavin (mg)	1.7	1.4	1.3	1.2
Niacin (mg)	19.0	15.0	15.0	13.0
Iron	–	–	15.0	10.0

*   RNI applies after 65 years
–   indicates values same for both age groups

may seem a strange decision, given the overwhelming evidence that average activity levels decline with age and thus so does the real ratio of energy expenditure to BMR (that is the real PAL almost certainly declines with age). The decision reflects the different priorities of the panel when dealing with younger and older adults. In the young, the panel has been keen to discourage overconsumption of energy (because of high levels of overweight and obesity) whilst in the elderly it has been keen to maintain sufficient energy intakes to allow adequate intakes of essential nutrients and to prevent people becoming underweight. These EARs are therefore likely to considerably understate the real decline in average energy intakes in the elderly. The US panel (NRC, 1989a) only gives energy allowances for those adults who are either over or under 50 years – the younger allowances are an estimated 1.60 times the Resting Energy Expenditure (REE) in men and 1.55 × REE in women, the older people's allowances are 1.50 times REE in men and women.

COMA (1992) quotes the results from a number of relatively small-scale surveys of the energy intakes of elderly people in the USA, Sweden and the UK. These studies are dated 1961–1980 and thus would not reflect recent declines in average intakes. The measured intakes in these studies varied from $1.25 \times$ BMR in a group of Swedish women (67–73 years) to $1.80 \times$ BMR in a very small group of elderly male crofters (active peasant farmers) in the north-west of Scotland (58–78 years). Such data underlines, once again, the heterogeneity of older people. Many, or perhaps most elderly people are very inactive and thus have low energy requirements but much of the fall in energy expenditure with age is probably avoidable.

Reference values for essential nutrients in the elderly

Table 5.2 (page 116) shows a comparison of the UK RNIs and US RDAs for elderly adults for several of the dietetically important essential nutrients. These values illustrate the level of disparity that can occur when different expert committees attempt to set dietary standards. The particular values represent expert opinion not scientific fact and expert opinions vary. In general the American values tend to be higher than the British ones and in some cases these differences are substantial (e.g. vitamin A, vitamin C, thiamin and zinc). Only in the case of vitamin D is the American value substantially below the UK RNI but in America this RDA is for all adults whereas the British RNI is only for the over 65s.

Table 5.3 shows how the US and UK dietary standards for older adults (over 50) differ from those given for younger adults – all values other than those listed are the same for the two groups. Thus the need for most nutrients is assumed to be the same in younger and older adults. This assumption has largely been made because of the absence of data upon which to quantify any possible differences, not because of clear evidence that the needs of young adults and the elderly are similar. The few small differences that are listed in Table 5.3 are explained as follows.

- Adult protein RNIs in the UK are calculated to represent 0.75 g protein/kg body weight per day and the small differences seen are solely due to differences in the average weights assumed for younger and older adults. As lean body mass and the ratio of lean to fat in the body decline with age, this protein RNI for older adults actually represents a higher protein intake per kilogram of *lean* tissue.
- B vitamin requirements are assumed to vary with total energy intake/expenditure and these standards have thus traditionally been set as amount of B vitamin per 1000 kcal of energy. Thus the UK thiamin RNIs are 0.4 mg of thiamin per 1000 kcal of the energy EAR for the group. Differing RNIs/RDAs for the B vitamins in the elderly are thus simply a reflection of the reduced energy EAR/RDA.
- The reduced iron RNI/RDA for elderly women reflects the reduced iron losses that result from the cessation of menstrual losses after the menopause.
- The UK panel assumed that for most adults under 65 years, endogenous production of vitamin D in the skin when exposed to sunlight was the primary source of the vitamin. Therefore, the RNI for vitamin D in older

adults (over 65) simply reflects the panel's view that this endogenous production can no longer be relied upon in elderly people who may be housebound and inadequately exposed to sunlight.

Thus with a few exceptions the requirements for essential nutrients in the elderly are not thought to be reduced. Energy requirements, on the other hand, are thought to decline and real intakes may often decline by substantially more than is suggested by the declining values shown in Table 5.1. COMA (1991) lists values of only 1.25 × BMR in some elderly Swedish women and COMA (1992) suggests that for many inactive elderly people, who only spend an hour a day on their feet, a value of 1.3 × BMR would represent their balance rather than the 1.5 × BMR used to set the EARs in COMA (1991). Thus elderly people are seen as requiring the same amounts of nutrients as younger adults, whilst they may well be consuming only about two-thirds the total amount of food. This makes it increasingly likely that, unless their diets are particularly rich in nutrients, they may satisfy their low energy needs whilst falling short of their requirements for other essential nutrients.

It is also possible that the absolute requirement for some nutrients may actually increase in old age, as that for dietary vitamin D is assumed to increase. Green (1994) suggests that some degree of malabsorption of several nutrients is probable in the elderly (see Chapter 3). The general conclusion of the UK panel on Dietary Reference Values (COMA, 1991), and the authors of an official UK report on nutrition in the elderly (COMA, 1992), was that there is little evidence for increased nutrient needs in the elderly with the exception of vitamin D. Poor nutrient status in the elderly is usually the result of poor intake or disease, rather than evidence of raised requirements. There is, however, a paucity of studies that have attempted to directly assess how nutrient requirements change with age; requirements for the elderly are usually derived by extrapolating from those of younger adults. There is also a general lack of satisfactory indices of nutritional status that have been directly tested and found to be reliable in the elderly. For example, a relatively large number of elderly Britons were found to have biochemical indications of riboflavin deficiency, using the criterion applied to younger people, but most had intakes of the vitamin that are considered satisfactory (DHSS, 1979). COMA (1991) specifically addresses this issue of how the needs of elderly adults differ from those of other adults for relatively few nutrients and their comments are summarised in the next section.

Specific references to changes in the requirement for nutrients with age in COMA (1991)

CALCIUM

There is reduced calcium absorption with age but this may be related to less efficient metabolism of vitamin D in the ageing kidney. (The conversion of vitamin D to its active form, 1,25-dihydroxycholecalciferol, occurs in the kidney and this active principle is necessary for the proper absorption of calcium in the intestine.) It recommended an increased allowance for vitamin D in the elderly, but felt that there was insufficient evidence to justify an increase in calcium intakes in those aged over 60 years.

VITAMIN B$_6$

There is a fall in the plasma concentration of the coenzyme derived from vitamin B$_6$ (pyridoxal phosphate) with age. The panel felt that there are probably changes in the absorption and metabolism of this vitamin with age and thus that the elderly may well have a higher absolute requirement. It felt, however, that there was insufficient evidence to quantify an increased RNI in the elderly.

VITAMIN B$_{12}$

There is a higher incidence of pernicious anaemia in the elderly. This is the disease that results from a failure to produce an intrinsic factor in the stomach that is necessary for vitamin B$_{12}$ absorption. It found no evidence, however, that healthy adult subjects had any increased *requirements* for vitamin B$_{12}$.

FOLATE

There is evidence of increased folate deficiency in the elderly but this is likely to be due to poor intake and it found no evidence of increased requirement in healthy elderly people. The elderly are also more likely to suffer from medical conditions that increase folate requirements.

VITAMIN C

Once again, it found no evidence for increased requirements in the elderly although elderly people often have low vitamin C status due to persistently low intakes.

Conclusions

There are large gaps in our knowledge of the nutritional requirements of older people. Nevertheless, this discussion of dietary standards for the elderly indicates that a number of practical measures could contribute to maintaining adequate intakes of essential nutrients in elderly people. The major problem that has to be addressed is the need to maintain intakes of essential nutrients despite a tendency for energy expenditure and total food intake to fall quite sharply as people become elderly.

- **There should be an emphasis on the need to on the need encourage and facilitate increased levels of activity in the population as a whole and**

reduce the decline in average activity levels with age. Increased levels of activity will have a direct effect on energy expenditure and thus raise energy and therefore probably nutrient intakes. Increased levels of activity are also likely to make an indirect contribution to increasing energy expenditure by maintaining the mass of metabolically active, lean tissue and thus reducing the normal age-related decline in BMR. Increased levels of activity in previously sedentary elderly people will probably result in increased muscle mass (e.g. Bassey, 1985; Fiatarone *et al.*, 1994). Increased activity, even at exercise loads well below those considered necessary to measurably affect aerobic fitness, will have many other benefits for older people (see Chapter 4).

- **Prevention of underweight should become an increasing priority as people get further into old age.** Low body weight reduces BMR and elderly people who are losing weight are not even meeting their reduced energy needs. Evidence was discussed in Chapter 4 (e.g. Campbell *et al.*, 1990; Mattela *et al*, 1986), that in the over 70s low body weight, low body fat and reduced lean mass may be much more significant predictors of mortality than overweight and obesity. Levels of overweight and obesity in the population peak in late middle age and are lower in the very elderly (see Table 4.1). To quote Exton-Smith (1988), 'the prognostic significance of being above average weight, which is adverse in younger persons, paradoxically becomes a favourable influence in the elderly'.

- **The need for high nutrient density of the diet should be an increasing priority as energy needs decline in old age** (nutrient density is the amount of nutrient per unit of energy in the diet, e.g. mg nutrient per kcal or kJ). A diet high in sugary or fatty foods, or alcoholic drinks, depresses the overall nutrient density of the diet because these things are high in energy but low in nutrients. Moderation of excessive alcohol intakes, reduced use of foods with added sugars and reduced use of high-fat foods should all contribute to increasing the nutrient density of elderly peoples' diets.

COMA (1992) recommends that elderly people, like the rest of the population, should be advised to eat more fresh vegetables, fruit and whole grain cereals. These changes are in line with the general dietary guidelines discussed in Chapter 4. Evidence from the *National Food Survey* (Table 1.10 and Table 4.11) suggests that the diets of elderly people may be particularly high in added sugars and this could therefore be a particular target area for nutrition education in the elderly. COMA (1992) suggests that in those sedentary elderly people whose energy expenditure is around 1.3 × BMR then 'the only means of ensuring nutrient intake is to have a low (below 10%) sugar intake'. *The National Food Survey* also indicates that absolute spending on fruits and vegetables is much lower in elderly households than in equivalent sized households of younger adults (see Table 1.10). Alcohol consumption is on average lower in older than younger adults although it may still be an important area of concern in a large minority of elderly people. More moderate use of added fats would probably contribute to increased nutrient density but some foods with an 'unhealthy fatty image' may be important sources of

Table 5.4 The micronutrient content of portions of some common foods expressed as a percentage of the UK RNI for an elderly man. Portion sizes are taken from Davies and Dickerson (1991) and individual items are medium sized

Vitamin A
Found as retinol in dairy fat, eggs, liver, fatty fish and supplemented foods like margarine. Found as carotene in many dark green, red or yellow fruits and vegetables.

1 cup whole milk	–	16%	40 g cheddar cheese	–	21%
90 g lamb liver	–	2643%	1 egg	–	16%
1 tomato	–	11%	95 g broccoli	–	57%
65 g carrots	–	186%	1 banana	–	4%
half cantaloup melon	–	100%	3 apricots (inc. canned)	–	36%
80 g fried cod roe	–	17%	5 g butter/margarine	–	6%
75 g frozen peas	–	5%	75 g spring greens	–	71%

Vitamin E (safe intake)
Found in vegetable oils, wheat germ and whole grain cereals, dark green leaves of vegetables, seeds and nuts.

1 egg	–	25%	5 g sunflower/olive/rapeseed oil	–	63/7/30%
1 slice wholemeal bread	–	1%	5 g butter/margarine	–	2.5/31%

Thiamin vitamin B_1
Found in all plant and animal tissues but only whole cereals, nuts, seeds and pulses are rich sources.

1 slice wholemeal bread(UK)	–	13%	1 egg	–	4%
1 pork chop	–	78%	1 cup whole milk	–	7%
30 g peanuts	–	30%	165 g brown/white rice	–	26/2%
75 g frozen peas	–	20%	200 g baked beans	–	16%
1 teaspoon (5 g) yeast extract	–	18%	150 g boiled potatoes	–	13%

Riboflavin – vitamin B_2
Small amounts in many foods, rich sources are liver, milk, cheese and egg.

1 slice wholemeal bread (UK)	–	2%	1 egg	–	16%
40 g cheddar cheese	–	12%	1 cup whole milk	–	25%
90 g lamb liver	–	308%	1 teaspoon (5 g) yeast extract	–	42%
95 g broccoli	–	15%	75 g frozen peas	–	4%
25 g corn flakes	–	19%	85 g canned sardines	–	18%

Niacin – vitamin B_3
Widely distributed in small amounts in many foods but good amounts in meat, offal, fish, wholemeal cereals and pulses; in some cereals, especially maize, much of the niacin may be as unavailable niacytin; the tryptophan in many food proteins is also a potential source of niacin. Values below are totals from both sources.

1 slice wholemeal bread (UK)	–	13%	90 g lamb liver	–	113%
1 pork chop	–	69%	95 g canned tuna	–	103%
1 egg	–	14%	1 cup whole milk	–	10%
75 g frozen peas	–	11%	25 g corn flakes	–	26%

Vitamin B$_6$ – pyridoxine
Liver is a rich source. Cereals, meats, fruits and vegetables all contain moderate amounts.

Vitamin B$_{12}$
Meat, fish, milk, eggs and fermented foods. In the UK meat substitutes are fortified.

Folic acid/folate
Liver, nuts, green vegetables and wholegrain cereals are good sources.

90 g lamb liver	–	110%	1 slice wholemeal bread (UK)	–	7%
peanuts	–	17%	95 g broccoli	–	50%
1 banana	–	15%	1 orange	–	45%
1 tspn (5 g) yeast extract	–	25%	25 g corn flakes	–	31%
75 g frozen peas	–	18%	75 g spring greens	–	25%

Vitamin C
Fruit, fruit juices together with salad and leafy vegetables are good sources.

95 g broccoli	–	75%	75 g frozen peas	–	25%
150 g boiled potatoes	–	35%	45 g sweet pepper		113%
1 tomato	–	38%	1 orange	–	238%
1 banana	–	20%	100 g strawberries	–	150%
1 apple	–	5%	200 ml orange juice	–	175%
1 glass 'Ribena' (blackcurrant cordial)	–	238%	200 ml tomato juice	–	100%

Potassium
Fruits and vegetables are the best sources; there is also some in milk, meat and fish.

1 orange	–	14%	1 banana	–	13%
1 apple	–	4%	95 g broccoli	–	6%
75 g frozen peas	–	3%	1 tomato	–	6%
265 g chips (F. fries)	–	77%	200 ml orange juice		7%

Zinc
Meats, whole grain cereals, pulses and shellfish are the main dietary sources of zinc.

1 slice wholemeal bread	–	7%	1 pork chop	–	30%
5 g frozen peas	–	5%	95 g lamb liver	–	42%
70 g canned crabmeat	–	37%			

Iron
Found in meat (particularly offal), fish, cereals and green vegetables. The biological availability of iron is much higher from meat and fish than from vegetable sources.

1 pork chop	–	11%	90 g lamb liver	–	103%
1 egg	–	13%	80 g peeled prawn	–	10%
85 g canned sardines	–	45%	75 g frozen peas	–	13%
95 g broccoli	–	11%	50 g bar of dark (plain) chocolate	–	14%
130 g spinach	–	60%	1 slice wholemeal bread	–	11%

nutrients, for example whole milk, cheese, eggs and meat. Table 5.4 shows some examples of the amounts of selected micronutrients in typical portions of common foods, expressed as a percentage of the UK RNI for an elderly man (the calcium and vitamin D content of some foods were given in Chapter 3 and the salt content of some foods in Chapter 4).

One cautionary note should be added at this point, if appetite is poor and/or the acuity of taste and smell are reduced there is a risk that changes in the diet that reduce its appeal and palatability may cause reduced intake and even weight loss; this could more than offset any theoretical benefits from the improved nutrient density.

The diets and nutritional status of elderly people

Sources of information

There is a general paucity of information about the nutritional status of the elderly in Britain and about what elderly non-institutionalised Britons eat. Many dietitians have undertaken weighed intakes and dietary assessments of elderly clients in the hospital setting. However, even this information has seldom been published in the scientific literature and has usually been confined to local use to modify meal provision and catering practices within the test hospital or district.

The lack of information about food intakes and nutritional status of elderly British people was highlighted in the COMA (1992) report *The nutrition of elderly people*. This COMA report makes frequent references to the results of a dietary and nutritional survey of 750 elderly, non-institutionalised British adults for which the fieldwork was carried out in 1967/68 (DHSS, 1972) and more especially a follow-up survey of 365 traceable survivors of the original sample five years later (DHSS, 1979). The most up to date, large, nationwide survey of the diets and nutritional status of elderly Britons is now nearly 30 years old. A large dietary and nutritional survey of a representative sample of elderly British adults is currently underway and is expected to be published in 1997 (Hughes *et al.*, 1995).

The 1967/68 survey of elderly British adults used a sample of 764 people living in six towns in England and Scotland (DHSS, 1972). Around 3% of the surveyed population were diagnosed as suffering from malnutrition and in about three-quarters of cases this malnutrition was associated with some precipitating medical condition. In the 1972/73 follow-up of the traceable survivors (DHSS, 1979) the subjects were then all over 70 years and the prevalence of malnutrition had risen to 7% with twice this frequency in subjects aged over 80 years. This longitudinal data indicates that the prevalence of malnutrition amongst the elderly UK population rises steeply with age. In both surveys, nutritional deficiencies were often related to some underlying disease; certain social factors were also strongly linked to the likelihood of being malnourished principally:

- immobility/being housebound
- social isolation
- living alone
- depression (e.g. associated with bereavement)
- low income
- low social class (IV and V)
- low mental test score.

Exton-Smith (1971) has identified six primary and six secondary causes of malnutrition in the elderly (summarised in Table 5.5)

One of the major conclusions of the 1972/73 survey was that, provided elderly people were in good general health, their diets were in general nature and types of food eaten, very similar to those of younger adults. This general conclusion has encouraged the belief that more recent surveys of the diets of younger adults (e.g. Gregory *et al.*, 1990) may also reflect the dietary patterns of elderly people (COMA, 1992). However, some indirect evidence has been presented in earlier chapters which suggests that there may be significant differences in the food purchases of younger and older adults in the UK. For example, in Figure 2.3 there is strong evidence that young and old may now differ quite markedly in their choice of cooking and spreading fats and in Table 1.10 and Table 4.11 there is a strong suggestion that the elderly may have relatively higher intakes of non-milk extrinsic sugars than younger adults. These subtle differences in the diets of younger and older adults may have important practical consequences and need to be clarified and quantified by direct studies of elderly people. Thus, for example, in its report on nutrition in the elderly, COMA (1992) accepts that intake of sugars in elderly Britons is probably towards the top end of the UK range (10–20%). The report goes on to suggest that the general dietary guidelines suggesting restriction of non-milk extrinsic sugars to 10% of total energy may be particularly important in the elderly because of the need to ensure a high nutrient density.

In the absence of a recent, large scale survey of the diets and nutritional status of elderly people in the UK, we have had to draw heavily upon the old data gathered in the 1972/73 survey of elderly Britons. We have supplemented this by use of small, often localised, surveys and surveys conducted in other countries to get a better picture of the likely current prevalence and types of nutritional problems in the elderly.

Total energy/food intake

The point has been made earlier in the chapter that low energy and low food intakes in the elderly increase the risk of concurrent vitamin and mineral deficiencies (COMA, 1992). It is generally accepted that the energy intakes of elderly people do tend to fall with advancing years for reasons discussed earlier in the chapter. Longitudinal data from the UK surveys of 1967/68 (DHSS, 1972) and 1972/73 (DHSS, 1979) indicated that energy intakes fell by an average of around 4% over this five year period. Sjogren *et al.* (1994) also found an

Table 5.5 Some causes of malnutrition in the elderly (after Exton-Smith, 1971)

Primary

Ignorance – at that time, many elderly people were ignorant of the basic facts of nutrition.

Social isolation – for example, the lack of interest in preparing food just for oneself, to eat alone; this issue was discussed in Chapter 2.

Physical disability – lack of mobility affects the ability to get and prepare food. Being housebound is a major precipitating factor for malnutrition in the elderly (DHSS, 1979).

Mental disturbances – confusion arising from degenerative states like dementia can precipitate malnutrition. Depressive conditions may lead to a lack of interest in preparing food and in eating.

Iatrogenic – malnutrition resulting from prolonged adherence to a poorly designed therapeutic diet e.g. a low acid diet used to treat gastric ulcer may lead to low intakes of vitamin C.

Poverty – the relative poverty of older people has been discussed in Chapter 1 and its possible effects on food choices and nutritional status have been discussed in Chapter 2.

Secondary

Impaired appetite – e.g. as a result of an infectious or other illness, drugs or radiotherapy, or simply the decline in taste and smell acuity with age.

Masticatory insufficiency – lack of teeth or ill fitting dentures was one of the factors that was identified in Chapter 2 as reducing the 'personal availability' of some foods to the elderly. See Chapter 3 for trends in dental health of the UK elderly.

Malabsorption – there is a general decrease in the efficiency of absorptive processes with age (Green, 1994). There is also an increased frequency of certain pathological conditions that substantially reduce the absorption of particular nutrients e.g. pernicious anaemia reduces vitamin B_{12} absorption.

Alcohol – alcohol displaces food from the diet and excessive intake reduces the absorption of some nutrients and increases some nutrient requirements.

Drugs – some drugs may affect nutrient absorption and metabolism e.g. folic acid metabolism may be affected by anti-convulsants. Some drugs may induce nausea or anorexia.

Increased requirements – there may be increased requirements for some nutrients in old age. As discussed earlier in the chapter, COMA (1991) felt that there was often insufficient evidence to specifically assess the nutritional requirements of older adults and these are usually extrapolated from the needs of other adults.

age-related decline in energy intakes in a six-year longitudinal study of a cohort of 70-year-old Swedes.

In the *Dietary and nutritional survey of British adults* (Gregory *et al.*, 1990), the sample was restricted to adults between 16 and 64 years but there was nevertheless a distinct trend towards decreasing energy intakes in the older age groups. The average intakes of 50- to 64-year-olds were significantly less than that of 35- to 49-year-olds: 5% less in men and 7% less in women. A Danish cross-sectional study of 1000 men and 1000 women in 1982–1984 found a marked decline in energy intakes across the age range 30–85 years. The average intake of 85-year-olds was only 72% of that of 30-year-olds in men and 79% in women (see Schroll et al., 1993).

Caughey et al. (1994) used an interview and 24 hour recall to assess the diets of 200 elderly people living in sheltered housing in Edinburgh. They found that energy intakes were lower in the over-75s as compared to those aged 65–74 years. About two-thirds of this sample had mean recorded intakes below the mean values recorded in the 1972/73 UK survey of elderly adults (DHSS, 1979) and about a fifth had intakes of less than 1200 kcal per day compared with the UK EARs for the over-65s that range from 1810–2330 kcal/day depending upon age and sex. At this very low intake of 1200 kcal/day, which for many subjects would be below their predicted BMR, there is a high risk of concurrent vitamin and mineral deficiency. Note, however, that the recall method used to determine food intake does tend to significantly underestimate real intakes.

Lewis et al. (1993) reported a small study of 20 elderly patients (mean age 76 years) attending a wound healing research centre for venous ulceration of the leg. The mean recorded energy intakes of this group were less than 1200 kcal/day which is again well below the EAR. Despite the very low recorded energy intakes, the mean body mass index of the sample was over 25. This apparent inconsistency could be due to very low energy expenditures in some subjects because they were rendered housebound or even bed-ridden by their leg ulcers (note also the possibility of underrecording). The authors of the study speculate upon whether this particular category of patients is, by the nature of their medical condition, more 'at risk' of nutritional inadequacy than other non-institutionalised elderly people. These results would seem to back-up the conclusion in the 1972/73 survey of elderly British people (DHSS, 1979) that being housebound is the most important social and medical risk factor predisposing to malnutrition in the elderly.

Vitamin C and the antioxidant vitamins

Data from the National Food Survey presented in Table 1.10 suggests that spending on fruits and vegetables is lower in OAP households than in other adult-only households; this difference widens still further if potatoes are excluded. In Table 4.11 this reduced spending on fruits and vegetables by OAP households is reflected in a slightly lower vitamin C content of purchased food and a substantially lower β-carotene content. Several sources suggest low intakes of fruits, fruit juices and cordials and vegetables in some elderly people. This would result in low intakes of not only vitamin C and carotene but also probably of folate, non-starch polysaccharide and potassium. Where elderly people derive a substantial proportion of their estimated vitamin C intake from institutionally catered meals (including meals on wheels and day centres), then real intakes may well be some way below estimated intakes because of the catering practices (e.g. prolonged warm-holding of food) that lead to large losses of vitamin C in the food before it is consumed. Low levels of leucocyte ascorbic acid (a biochemical measure of vitamin C status) have also been reported in the elderly by many groups of workers. These low levels do indicate nutritional adequacy and are not simply a natural accompaniment to ageing since they can be raised to levels found in the young by ascorbic acid feeding (Exton-Smith, 1988).

The 1972/73 survey of elderly UK adults (DHSS, 1979) found that more than half of the sample had intakes of vitamin C that are below the present UK RNI of 40 mg/day. In their survey in Edinburgh, Caughey et al. (1994) reported that 90% of the residents of the surveyed population living in sheltered accommodation never drank vitamin C enriched squashes or cordials or fruit juices. Lewis et al. (1993) found that although mean intakes of vitamin C in their small sample of leg ulcer patients were above the UK RNI, nevertheless several individuals had very low intakes. Most of the vitamin C consumed by this sample came from potatoes with very little obtained from fruit or fruit juices.

Newton et al. (1985) found low intakes of vitamin C and low blood concentrations in a sample of chronically sick, elderly American women. They confirmed that the low blood concentrations were primarily the result of poor intake because small dietary supplements increased concentrations of vitamin C in both plasma and leucocytes.

Penn et al. (1991) investigated some of the consequences of poor antioxidant vitamin status in elderly people. They allocated 30 elderly, long stay patients to receive either dietary supplements of vitamins A,C and E or a placebo for a period of 28 days. Nutritional status and cell-mediated immune function were assessed before and after the period of supplementation. Following vitamin supplementation, measures of the cell-mediated immune function improved and there was a significant increase in the absolute number of T-cells. In contrast, no significant changes were noted in the immune function of the placebo group. They conclude that dietary antioxidants – vitamins A, C and E – can improve aspects of cell-mediated immune function in elderly long-stay patients and should be considered as a possible intervention.

B vitamins

In the 1972/73 survey of elderly UK adults, 30% of the sample had biochemical indices of riboflavin status that are usually taken to be less than satisfactory, that is they had an erythrocyte glutathione reductase activation coefficient (EGRAC) of greater than 1.3 (see Chapter 6 for more information on the EGRAC). However, there was no indication of similarly high numbers of elderly people having intakes of riboflavin below the current RNI. There is some confusion about the relationship between biochemical indices of riboflavin status and dietary intake. Non-dietary factors may have a substantial effect upon riboflavin status, particularly in the elderly (COMA, 1992). Riboflavin status is likely to be very dependent upon milk consumption, as milk and milk products supply more than a quarter of the riboflavin in the diets of UK adults under 65 years; breakfast cereals, which are often fortified, supply a further 10% of UK riboflavin intakes (Gregory *et al.*, 1990).

There may be increased prevalence of vitamin B_{12} deficiency in the elderly because of increased incidence of diseases that hinder absorption rather than due to dietary inadequacy *per se*. Requirements for vitamin B_{12} are minute (see Table 5.2) but efficient absorption of B_{12} requires the presence of an intrinsic factor secreted by the parietal cells in the stomach. Pernicious anaemia is an autoimmune disease which leads to failure of intrinsic factor production and thus to B_{12} deficiency. The symptoms of B_{12} deficiency are a severe mega-loblastic anaemia and neurological manifestations including an irreversible and progressive degeneration of the spinal cord. Gastrectomy and gastric atrophy in the elderly will impair intrinsic factor production and B_{12} absorp-tion. Reduced absorptive capacity in the small intestine where the B_{12} is absorbed can also reduce B_{12} status; this reduced absorptive capacity occurs both as a general consequence of ageing and as a consequence of some age-related intestinal diseases. In the 1972/73 survey of elderly people, only around 2.5% had biochemical indices of B_{12} status that are considered to be abnormal but a further 18% had levels considered to be at the borderline of adequacy. As already stated, COMA (1991) accepted that increased prevalence of diseases that impair absorption do occur in the elderly but they concluded that there was no compelling evidence for an increased dietary requirement for B_{12} in healthy, elderly people. Vitamin B_{12} is generally found only in foods of animal origin (meat, fish and milk); it is however also present in fermented foods and many vegetarian foods are fortified with B_{12} in the UK.

DHSS (1979) found that in 1972/73 only about 5% of their sample of elder-ly people had biochemical indices of folate status that are considered to be abnormal, although about a quarter had borderline levels. Vegetables and offal are prime dietary sources of folate.

Intakes of thiamin in elderly people recorded in the 1972/73 UK survey were only about half those reported in the 1986/87 survey of 16–64-year-old British adults by Gregory *et al.*, 1990. In the elderly sample, 8% had biochem-ical indices of thiamin status outside the range considered to be satisfactory (that is 8% had erythrocyte transketolase activation coefficients above 1.25). Almost 40% of the thiamin in the diets of younger adults comes from cereal products, especially from bread and breakfast cereals (white bread and many breakfast cereals are fortified with thiamin). Potatoes and meat each provide about 20% of the thiamin in these UK diets (Gregory *et al.*, 1990).

Vitamin D

There has already been substantial discussion of the vitamin D requirements and the vitamin D status of elderly people both earlier in this chapter and in Chapter 3 in the section dealing with the ageing skeleton. The principal source of vitamin D in most adults is endogenous production in the skin when it is exposed to summer sunlight. UK dietary intakes are only around 2 µg per day and this is well below levels considered necessary to produce satisfactory vitamin D status in the absence of skin production (5–10 μg per day). There is evidence of unsatisfactory vitamin D status amongst the elderly UK population, particularly in the winter months and primarily in those elderly people who are housebound or get limited exposure to summer sunshine (Thurnham, 1992; COMA, 1991).

Minerals

CALCIUM

The relationship between calcium intake, vitamin D status and bone health has been discussed in Chapter 3. Accordingly it would seem prudent to ensure that the calcium intakes of elderly people are in line with those seen in the DRVs in Table 5.2. Almost half of UK dietary calcium (in those under 65 years) comes from milk and milk products; this is also the best absorbed source of dietary calcium. Elderly people need to maintain good intakes of milk.

IRON

Iron deficiency anaemia is the most common of the micronutrient deficiency diseases in both developed and developing countries. Young women are recognised as a high risk group because of iron losses in menstrual blood and iron losses associated with childbearing. Iron deficiency results in a microcytic anaemia because iron is essential for the synthesis of the oxygen transporting pigment, haemoglobin, that makes up about 85% of the dry weight of red blood cells. Symptoms of tiredness, lack of energy, breathlessness upon exertion and palpitations are commonly associated with anaemia. The relationship between dietary iron intake and iron status is not straightforward for several reasons, as listed below.

- Any state that results in chronic blood loss increases the risk of iron deficiency because it increases iron losses, e.g. menstruation, haemorrhoids (piles), some cancers, peptic ulcer, chronic use of aspirin-type drugs.
- There is very great variation in the availability of dietary iron from different sources. Iron from meat and fish is much better absorbed than that from most vegetable sources.
- Some other dietary components may promote or inhibit the absorption of iron; vitamin C and alcohol promote absorption whereas bran and the tannin in tea hinder absorption.
- Some conditions affect the efficiency of iron absorption. For example, any condition that reduces gastric acid production will reduce the efficiency of iron absorption; these conditions are more prevalent in the elderly.
- The efficiency of iron absorption is influenced by iron status; when iron stores are full, iron absorption is less 'efficient' than when they are depleted.

Thus elderly people are more likely to be affected by a variety of conditions that may increase iron losses and reduce the efficiency of iron absorption. Low intake of vitamin C, which has been found in many elderly people, would also adversely affect the efficiency of iron absorption.

Blood haemoglobin concentration has been the traditional biochemical measure of iron status, although it is now regarded as both an insensitive and a non-specific measure of iron status. For example, there may be considerable depletion of iron stores before there is any significant fall in blood haemoglobin concentration and blood haemoglobin concentration is affected by things other than simply iron status: things such as altitude, exercise level and renal disease. A level of 12 g Hb/dl has traditionally been taken as the level below which there is increasing likelihood of anaemia. In a survey of English adults, White *et al.* (1993) found that 17% of men and 39% of women aged over 75 years had haemoglobin levels below 12.5 g/dl and about 10% of the over 75s had levels below 11 g/dl. Haemoglobin concentrations of less than 11 g/dl are very uncommon in young men and even in women only about 4% of the total sample (aged 16+ years) had haemoglobin concentrations of less than 11 g/dl, although about a third had levels below 12.5 g/dl. Ferritin is the major storage form of iron in the body and serum ferritin is now regarded as a more sensitive and specific indicator of iron status; values of less than 13 µg/l are taken to indicate subnormal iron status and those in the range 13–25 µg/l are regarded as marginal. White *et al.* (1993) found that, in their sample of English adults, average serum ferritin levels tended to rise with age up to about 65 years in men and 75 years in women whereafter they fell away. In the over 75 age group 6% of men and 12% of women had values that indicated subnormal iron status and a further 9% of men and 11% of women had values in the marginal range. Figure 5.3 shows how the measured iron status of the over 75s in a large English sample compares to that of the population as a whole.

Studies of elderly, hospitalised patients indicate that their iron intakes are lower than those of apparently healthy, independent, elderly people. This is almost entirely as a result of reduced caloric intake; the nutrient densities of the two diets were very similar for iron (COMA, 1992). Once again, there is

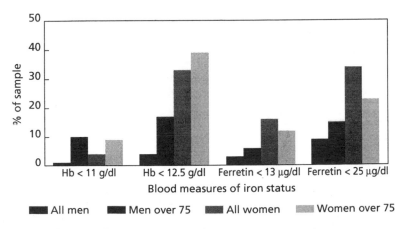

Figure 5.3 Iron status in young and old. Source: White *et al.* (1993)

seen to be a need for increased nutrient density if energy intakes fall but nutrient requirements do not.

Average intakes of iron in UK adults aged 16–64 years are 12.3 mg/day in men and 10.5 mg/day in women. These values are both comfortably in excess of the current UK RNI for elderly people (8.7 mg/day). Iron intakes are, however, not normally distributed, with substantial numbers of people with very high intakes (over three times the average) or very low intakes (less than half the average. About a quarter of iron in the diets of these younger adult Britons comes from meat and fish and this is the best absorbed source of dietary iron. Cereals provide 42% of the iron in British diets and this is likely to be relatively poorly absorbed whilst vegetables provide about 15% of total iron and the availability of this iron may be increased by the presence of vitamin C in the vegetables.

ZINC

Zinc deficiency is associated with impaired cell mediated immune responses and with reduced wound healing. In zinc deficient subjects, supplements can lead to improvements in these parameters (COMA, 1992). There is little to suggest that zinc deficiency is a particular problem for healthy, independent elderly people in the UK (COMA, 1992) although in Table 4.11 there is just a hint of slightly lower zinc intakes in older adults.

The nutritional status of elderly hospital patients

Hospital malnutrition – the general problem

In her *Notes on nursing*, published in the middle of the last century, Florence Nightingale recognised that there was a high prevalence of malnutrition amongst hospital patients and that this was often the result of inadequate care:

> *Thousands of patients are annually starved in the midst of plenty, from want of attention to the ways which alone make it possible for them to take food.*

In the mid 1970s, reports emanating from both the USA (e.g. Bistrian *et al.*, 1974) and the UK (e.g. Hill *et al.*, 1977), refocused attention upon this problem of hospital malnutrition by reporting very high prevalence of malnutrition amongst random samples of surgical patients. They not only reported high prevalence of malnutrition but also noted an almost complete lack of attention to assessing and monitoring the nutritional status of patients – Hill *et al.* found that only 15% of the patients in their survey had been weighed at any time during their stay in hospital.

Other studies have looked more directly at the adequacy of the food consumed by hospital patients. Todd *et al.* (1984) monitored the food consumed over a five-day period by a sample of 55 hospital patients from four different

Table 5.6 Factors that may contribute towards poor nutritional status in hospital patients (modified after Webb, 1995)

1   Physical difficulties with eating, for example: difficulties in swallowing; arthritis; and diseases affecting co-ordination and motor functions. Such problems may be particularly prevalent amongst very elderly patients.

2   Malabsorption of nutrients due to disease of the alimentary tract. Some malabsorptive conditions become more prevalent with age and there is a general age-related decline in absorptive efficiency in the gut.

3   Anorexia induced by treatment or disease.

4   Anorexia resulting from a psychological response to illness, hospitalisation or diagnosis.

5   Unacceptability and poor nutritional quality of hospital food. Lack of choice, prolonged warm-holding of food and simply unfamiliarity may all further reduce nutrient intake in people whose appetite may already be impaired.

6   Unavailability of food. Periods of enforced starvation for surgery and tests are obvious general factors here. Inadequate time allowed for meals, lack of help with eating and poor spacing of meals may be factors that particularly affect some elderly people. Staff may well underestimate the needs of elderly patients and provide inadequate amounts of food.

7   Increased nutrient losses, e.g. from wounds, urinary losses of glucose in elderly diabetic patients or urinary protein losses in elderly renal patients.

8   Increased nutrient turnover in some patients – febrile illness and injury lead to hypermetabolism. Paradoxically the energy needs of some elderly, immobile and wasted patients may be so low as to make inadequacy of other nutrients probable.

areas of a hospital. The average energy intakes of a quarter of these patients was less than their predicted metabolic rates and many patients had daily intakes of iron and vitamins that were below the then UK RDAs for healthy adults. Illness is frequently associated with a lack of appetite and poor food and nutrient intake. Webb (1995) has previously listed a number of factors that might contribute to the poor nutritional intakes and status of sick and injured patients and these are summarised in Table 5.6.

In 1992, the King's Fund Centre published a report entitled *A positive approach to nutrition* as treatment (KFC, 1992). From a review of the literature, they concluded that up to 50% of surgical patients and up to 44% of medical patients are malnourished on admission to hospital. Whilst many patients are malnourished on admission to hospital there is also a general tendency for nutritional status to decline during hospitalisation. KFC (1992) concluded that 'many people with severe illness are at risk from an unrecognised complication – malnutrition' and that 'doctors and nurses frequently fail to recognise under-nourishment because they are not trained to look for it'. These conclusions are disturbingly similar to those quoted from Florence Nightingale's writings of 125 years ago.

The King's Fund report suggested that malnutrition amongst hospital patients was associated with increased rates of complications, higher mortality rates, increased duration of hospital stay and thus also increased costs. More specifically they suggested that malnutrition leads to ...

- **higher rates of wound infections.** Malnutrition is known to cause large decreases in several measures of immunocompetence (Chandra, 1993); cell-mediated immune function is particularly depressed. Ageing also leads to decreased immunocompetence (discussed in Chapter 3). The consequences of malnutrition and ageing *per se* may compound in depressing the immune function of elderly patients.
- **increased risk of general infections** partly as a consequence of the reduced immunocompetence. Malnourished patients may be particularly prone to respiratory infections and pneumonia because weakening of the respiratory muscles will impair the ability to cough and expectorate. Once again, both ageing and malnutrition are associated with a decline in muscle strength and respiratory function.
- **increased risk of pressure sores** because of wasting and immobility. Lean body mass declines in old age and the prevalence of low body weight increases in old age (Table 4.1). Ageing is itself associated with reduced mobility and decreased circulatory efficiency.
- **increased risk of thromboembolism** because of immobility.
- **increased liability to heart failure** because of wasting and reduced function of cardiac muscle. In Figure 3.1 in Chapter 3, a decline in cardiac output with age is seen: the output in an 80-year-old is typically only about two-thirds of that in a 20-year-old.
- **increased likelihood of a range of adverse psychological conditions** as a consequence of starvation (e.g. apathy and depression).

Despite publications like those cited above and presumably heightened awareness of malnutrition in hospital patients, the situation in the UK would not seem to have improved to any major extent since the 1970s. In a recent re-examination of the problem, McWhirter and Pennington (1994) found that 40% of a sample of 100 consecutive admissions to each of five separate areas of an acute teaching hospital in the UK were undernourished upon admission. Most of the 500 patients lost weight during their hospital stay and weight loss was greatest in those patients who were most undernourished on admission. Those small number of patients referred for nutritional support (obviously amongst the most severely malnourished at admission), showed an average weight gain during their stay. This would strongly indicate that the undernourishment recorded at admission is usually reversible and also that much of the worsening of nutritional status that is frequently associated with hospitalisation can be avoided with appropriate care. In the 100 patients in the 'medicine for the elderly' speciality in this survey, the rate of undernutrition at admission was comparable to that in the overall sample at 43%. In studies that have specifically looked at elderly patients, high rates of undernutrition upon admission and a tendency for nutritional status to deteriorate during admission have been general findings. They have been reported in acutely ill elderly patients (Klipstein-Grobusch *et al.*, 1995), long stay geriatric patients (Morgan *et al.*, 1986; Larsson *et al.*, 1990), psychogeriatric patients

(Prentice *et al.*, 1989) and patients admitted for specific problems such as hip fractures (Bastow *et al.*, 1983).

Malnutrition amongst hospital patients seems to be a general problem found in most hospital specialities ranging from medical to surgical patients and from paediatric to geriatric patients (KFC, 1992). However, the elderly do make up a disproportionately large sector of the hospital population and the consequences of malnutrition may be greater in the elderly because they are likely to compound with some of the general deterioration in physiological functioning with age such as is discussed in Chapter 3.

Nutritional status of the elderly in hospital

Table 5.7 shows a summary of the findings of six papers that have reported upon the nutrient intakes of elderly hospital patients. There has been a consistent tendency for these studies to report low intakes of energy and most studies have also noted low intakes of vitamin C, vitamin D, folate and iron. Note that a failure to record low intakes of particular nutrients in this table may be because they were not measured rather than that intake was found to be satisfactory.

Jones *et al.* (1988) assessed the nutrient intake of 90 elderly (average age 83 years), long stay, female patients who had been hospitalised for more than three months and who were mostly suffering from either strokes or Parkinson's disease. They were particularly interested in the vitamin C content of the ingested food and this was determined by analysis of representative

Table 5.7 Energy and nutrient deficiencies recorded in six studies of elderly hospital patients

Nutrient	Brown (1991)	Kirk (1990)	Simon (1991)	Fenton (1989)	Jones et al. (1988)	Prior (1992)
Energy	Low	Low	Low	Low	Low	Low
Protein			Low		Low	
Fibre	Low	Low	Low			Low
Vitamin C	Low	Low	Low	Low	Low	Low
Vitamin D	Low	Low	Low	Low		Low
Folate	Low	Low	Low	Low		Low
Iron	Low	Low	Low	Low		
Zinc	Low					Low
Calcium	Low		Low			

NB Failure to find low intake may be because the nutrient was not measured.

samples of the plated meals just prior to serving. Vitamin C intake was on average only 17 mg/day (UK RNI is 40 mg/day and USA RDA is 60 mg/day). These intakes were less than those recorded in other studies where vitamin C intake has been determined using standard food tables. The extended warm-holding of food prior to serving was an important factor in the low intakes of these patients; food often remained in the trolleys for well over an hour before being served to patients. Only vitamin C was measured, but the authors suggest that the low vitamin C intakes might indicate generally low intakes of the water soluble vitamins. Plate waste, particularly of vitamin C-fortified mashed potato was another factor that reduced the vitamin C intakes of these patients. The mean energy intakes of these very immobile patients was only 1140 kcal/day which is around the expected BMR for women of this age. With such low intakes of food energy the concurrent risk of other nutrient inadequacies must be high.

Kirk (1990) assessed the nutrient content of food served to and consumed by a small group of elderly patients in a long stay hospital for the elderly. Patients in this study were served meals that contained less than 90% of the estimated energy requirements of healthy elderly people and actually consumed less than 90% of the food they were offered. Intakes of not only energy but also fibre, iron, vitamin C, vitamin D and folate were considered to be inadequate. Kirk also identified several factors in the nursing and catering practices that were likely to have had an adverse impact upon food and nutrient intake; these have been incorporated into the list in Table 5.8. Chapter 7 deals with ways in which the nutritional status of elderly people, including elderly hospital patients, could be improved.

Table 5.8 Some service provision factors that may depress food and nutrient intakes in elderly hospital patients (or clients in residential and nursing homes)

1   Timing of meals. In many hospitals, meals are bunched together during the working day with long enforced fasts from early evening to morning.
2   Prolonged holding of food prior to serving leads to deterioration of both nutritional quality and palatability.
3   Inherently unappetising food and limited choice.
4   Failure to allow choice – Kirk (1990) found that some elderly patients who were capable of making their own choices from the menu, nonetheless had choices made for them by staff.
5   Providing patients with portions of food that are insufficient for their needs sometimes because of staff underestimation of the needs of elderly patients.
6   Plate wastage not monitored or recorded by staff and so very low intakes are not recognised early.
7   Inadequate amount of time allowed for slow feeders to finish their meals.
8   Lack of staff help and/or feeding aids for those who need help with eating. Staff shortages may mean that even where help is provided, by the time it is forthcoming, the food is cold and even more unappetising.

Drugs and nutritional status in the elderly

Elderly people take more medicines than younger adults. In the USA, the over 65s account for a quarter of all the prescribed and over-the-counter drugs sold. In a 1984 survey less than 40% of elderly people in England had not taken at least one prescribed medicine in the 24 hours before interview; almost a quarter of them had taken three or more prescribed medicines. The most common types of prescribed drugs in this survey were diuretics, hypnotics and sedatives, β-blockers, analgesics and aspirin, and drugs for the treatment of rheumatism and gout (DH, 1992a). But these prescribed medicines probably represent only about 40% of the total medicines consumed by older people, the other 60% being over-the-counter preparations such as analgesics, antacids and laxatives. Prescribed and over-the-counter drugs may affect nutritional status and conversely diet and nutritional status can affect the functioning of drugs. The interactions between drugs and nutrition is thus a topic that has particular importance to the elderly.

Effect of nutrition upon drugs

Ageing results in a reduction in lean body mass, a reduced ability to metabolise drugs and a decline in renal function and thus a decline in the ability to excrete drugs. The marginal nutritional inadequacies frequently seen in older people will also impair their ability to metabolise drugs. These factors compound to increase the sensitivity of older people to drugs and make them more prone to drug toxicity. Some examples of the effects of food and nutritional status upon the absorption, metabolism and excretion of drugs are given below; further details may be found in Dickerson (1988), Roe (1993) and Cataldo et al. (1995).

CATABOLISM OF DRUGS

The hepatic mixed oxidase enzyme system is of key importance in the metabolism and detoxification of many drugs and other ingested chemicals. The activity of this system, and its induceability, decline with age and is also reduced by general undernutrition and by several micronutrient deficiencies. Ageing and malnutrition have a compounding effect in reducing the rate of metabolism of many drugs.

ABSORPTION OF DRUGS

Some nutrients may affect the absorption of drugs from the gut – some are better absorbed when taken with food and some when taken on an empty stomach. For example:

- calcium in milk binds with the antibiotic tetracyline and reduces its absorption
- food in the stomach slows down the rate of aspirin absorption (but food also lessens the gastric irritation caused by aspirin)
- some dietary amino acids can hinder the absorption of L-dopa (used in the

treatment of Parkinson's disease) by competing with binding sites in the intestine.

INTERACTION BETWEEN DRUGS AND NUTRIENTS

Some nutrients and drugs interact metabolically. For example:

- some anticoagulants (e.g. warfarin) work by blocking the action of vitamin K; the effects of the drugs are reversed by high intakes of vitamin K
- some anti-depressants (monoamine oxidase inhibitors) sensitise people to the effects of the substance tyramine present in foods like red wine, ripe cheese, smoked fish and broad beans – such foods can cause a dangerous rise in blood pressure in people taking these drugs.

EXCRETION OF DRUGS

Foods can affect the rate of excretion of drugs (note also the age-related decline in renal function which decreases the renal excretion of many drugs). For example, high doses of vitamin C make urine acidic and reduce the excretion of aspirin.

Effect of drugs upon nutrition

Drugs have the potential to affect nutritional status: they can have effects upon the intake, absorption, utilisation or excretion of nutrients by a variety of mechanisms, including those listed below.

EFFECTS ON FOOD INTAKE

Drugs can affect food intake. There may be direct effects upon the brain mechanisms regulating appetite or other effects that will indirectly affect food intake, e.g. altering taste and smell, producing nausea, causing irritation in the gastrointestinal tract or simply by causing a dry mouth. For example:

- the biguanide oral antidiabetics depress appetite and this may be an advantage of their use in overweight and obese elderly diabetics
- the other major category of oral antidiabetic agents, the sulphonylureas, increase appetite and weight gain and this will tend to exacerbate the obesity of many older diabetics and further decrease their sensitivity to insulin
- several of the cytotoxic drugs used in cancer chemotherapy have an anorectic effect, tending to depress food intake and cause further weight loss in patients who may already be underweight because of the effects of their disease
- antidepressants may increase appetite and weight gain in previously depressed patients and likewise tranquilizers in patients with anxiety states
- alcohol can substitute for other food and thus depress the intake of nutrients generally and nutritional inadequacy is a common feature of chronic alcohol abuse

- small amounts of alcohol may have a stimulating effect upon appetite in sick people
- phenobarbital can cause a dry mouth.

EFFECTS ON ABSORPTION

Drugs can alter the absorption of nutrients. For example:

- cytoxic drugs used in cancer chemotherapy can cause damage to the intestinal mucosa and precipitate multiple nutrient deficiencies due to malabsorption
- alcohol reduces the absorption of thiamin; the neurological symptoms of thiamin deficiency (Wernicke-Korsakoff syndrome) are frequently seen in alcoholics.

EFFECTS ON EXCRETION

Drugs can alter the rate of excretion or metabolism of nutrients. For example:

- diuretics can increase the excretion of potassium and sodium.

Further examples of particular drugs or groups of drugs that are likely to be taken by elderly people and that are believed to affect the status of patients for particular nutrients are shown in Table 5.9.

Table 5.9 Some effects of drugs upon nutrient status. Data sources: Dickerson (1988) and Roe (1993)

Drugs	Nutrient	Effect of drug
Laxatives (mineral oil)	Potassium Fat soluble vitamins	Depletion Malabsorption
Aspirin	Iron	Increases loss due to gastric bleeding
Corticosteroids	Protein Vitamin C	Depletion – loss of bone and muscle Increases excretion
Bile acid sequesters (e.g. cholestyramine)	Fat soluble vitamins	Malabsorption
Anticonvulsants	Folic acid Vitamin D	Reduced absorption Precipitates signs of deficiency
Tetracycline	Vitamin C	Increases excretion
Antacids	Phosphate Iron	Decreases absorption Decreases absorption?
Thiazide diuretics	Potassium	Depletion

6 Nutritional assessment and screening in the elderly

Aims and scope of the chapter

'Nutritional assessment' could be defined as observations and measurements that make it possible to judge a person's nutritional state. 'Medical screening' is usually taken to mean a process of identifying previously undiagnosed clinical or subclinical disease or identifying those who are at increased risk of developing a particular disease. In the context of this book, the term 'screening' is used more widely to also include identification of those with disability, malnutrition or with social/economic/environmental circumstances that may precipitate malnutrition or illness. The nutritional assessment methods described in the first part of the chapter, clearly have their place in screening the elderly population. However, as medical and socioeconomic factors are frequently linked to malnutrition (DHSS, 1979), then methods of assessing these factors may also play a major part in many nutritional screening tools.

Identification of nutritional problems should make it possible to design appropriate and relevant interventions to improve nutritional status. Nutritional assessment methods are designed to identify specific biological problems such as undernutrition, obesity and vitamin/mineral deficiencies. The causes of the problem then need to be identified and this usually simplifies the decision about what is the most effective and appropriate intervention. Intervention may take the form of dietary advice, changes in catering practices, social support, meal or supplement provision, and/or medical treatment. Some examples of the diverse causes of nutritional problems are:

- poor catering practices, such as prolonged warm holding of vegetables, may precipitate vitamin C deficiency
- chronic blood loss from an ulcer or as a consequence of intestinal cancer may be the cause of poor iron status
- reduced mobility may hinder someone's ability to shop and prepare food and thus precipitate malnutrition
- lack of exposure to sunlight in an elderly housebound person may be the cause of their poor vitamin D status
- inadequate time allowed for meals or lack of help with eating may lead to undernutrition in residential homes and hospitals
- intellectual deterioration as the result of dementia may lead to inadequate food intake and malnutrition.

The aims of this chapter are threefold:

- to review the specific clinical, anthropometric, biochemical and dietary methods used in nutritional assessment, in particular, their application and appropriateness for older people and the availability of reliable standards for older people
- to outline briefly the requirements for mandatory general screening of all patients over 75 years that is now written into the contracts of general practitioners working within the UK National Health Service; we will consider the philosophy behind this screening, its aims, its practice and the potential place for nutritional screening within this general framework
- to review some of the simple screening tools that have been designed to try to produce a cheap and quick method of identifying those individuals suffering from or at risk of malnutrition, either in the community or in an institutional setting. In addition to screening individuals, some screening tools seek to identify institutional practices that lead to increased risk of malnutrition amongst residents.

Methods of nutritional assessment

Observations and clinical signs

Deficiency of a nutrient will ultimately lead to a clinically apparent deficiency disease which often has well-defined signs and symptoms. For example, vitamin C deficiency ultimately leads to the disease scurvy which is characterised by symptoms such as bleeding gums, subdermal haemorrhages, impaired wound healing and a tendency for scar tissue to break down. However, these clinical signs of deficiency usually only become apparent as the end result of a prolonged and/or severely inadequate intake so that their absence does not necessarily guarantee satisfactory nutrient status. They tend to be very insensitive indicators of nutritional problems and are therefore not useful as early warning of dietary/nutritional problems. Many of the clinical signs of deficiency are also non-specific; the same symptom may be present in several deficiency states and may also be of non-nutritional origin. For example, oedema occurs in protein-energy malnutrition, some cases of beriberi, heart failure, liver disease, renal disease and many other circumstances.

Despite their lack of sensitivity and specificity, these clinical signs are useful because they can be picked up by any vigilant person who is in contact with elderly people and who knows what signs to look for; it does not require specialist equipment or highly trained personnel to detect them. The baggy appearance of clothing or a loose fitting belt would be strong indications of recent weight loss and would be apparent to any vigilant observer. Some outward signs and symptoms that may indicate a nutritional problem are listed in Table 6.1.

The COMA (1992) report on the nutrition of elderly people recommended that further research was needed to clarify the clinical features of nutrient deficiencies and it specifically listed the B vitamins, vitamin D, zinc and copper.

Table 6.1 Signs and symptoms that may indicate malnutrition or a nutrient deficiency in elderly people

Loose, hanging clothes may indicate recent weight loss
Wasted appearance and lack of subcutaneous fat
Oedema
Enlarged liver
Pale conjunctiva
Angular stomatitis – spongy lesions at the corners of the mouth
Cheilosis – a red, inflamed area at the line of closure of the lips
Glossitis – raw, inflamed tongue
Spongy, bleeding gums
Petechiae – small red blotches caused by subdermal haemorrhages
Spontaneous bruising
Some types of dermatitis
Muscle wasting
Loss of sensation at periphery
Listlessness, apathy and/or confusion
Spoon shaped fingernails (koilonychia)

Note that several of these symptoms have non-nutritional causes that may even be the more likely cause

Anthropometric measures

These are physical measurements of body size and dimensions; they are collectively the most used and most useful indicators of nutritional status. Although they vary in the ease and accuracy with which they can be measured, they are all quantitative measures and their usefulness is very dependent upon the availability of reliable and validated standards. Table 6.2 shows the 5th, 50th and 95th percentiles according to age band of several

Table 6.2 Anthropometric norms for elderly people based on large samples of Welsh (Burr and Phillips, 1984) and English elderly people (White *et al.*, 1993)

Data of Burr and Phillips (1984)

Measure/percentile		Age groups (years)				
		65–69	70–74	75–79	80–84	85+
BMI (kg/m²)						
5th	♂	18.1	18.9	17.5	18.1	17.0
	♀	17.2	18.4	18.1	17.1	16.7
50th	♂	24.3	25.1	23.9	23.7	23.1
	♀	26.5	26.3	26.1	25.5	23.6
95th	♂	30.5	31.3	30.3	29.3	28.4
	♀	33.8	32.4	32.4	32.0	29.0
MAC (mm)						
5th	♂	206	209	197	193	189
	♀	212	201	193	179	164
50th	♂	260	255	245	237	230
	♀	264	255	249	235	221
95th	♂	314	301	293	281	271
	♀	317	309	305	291	278
Triceps (mm)						
5th	♂	3.6	3.7	3.6	3.5	3.4
	♀	9.9	8.2	7.5	6.2	6.0
50th	♂	8.1	8.0	7.0	6.6	6.5
	♀	18.0	15.9	14.6	12.7	11.5
95th	♂	18.2	17.3	13.6	12.3	12.2
	♀	32.5	31.1	28.4	26.2	21.8
MAMC (mm)						
5th	♂	187	184	182	176	172
	♀	163	158	161	151	141
50th	♂	231	227	221	215	208
	♀	204	201	200	192	182
95th	♂	275	270	260	254	244
	♀	245	244	239	233	223

Table 6.2 (continued) Data of White *et al.* (1993):

Measure/percentile	Age band (years)			
	65–74	65–74	75+	75+
BMI (kg/m²)	♂	♀	♂	♀
5th	21.0	19.7	19.7	19.0
50th	26.0	26.3	25.2	25.2
95th	32.9	33.7	32.5	33.7
Mindex (kg/m)				
5th	77.2	66.0	69.2	63.0
50th	94.0	88.5	92.2	85.3
95th	115.4	114.6	115.1	116.1
Demiquet (kg/m²)				
5th	93.6	87.9	85.3	85.6
50th	114.9	119.9	112.6	117.7
95th	145.5	160.1	141.4	164.6

commonly used anthropometric measures in large samples of elderly Welsh or English men and women (Burr and Phillips, 1984; White *et al.*, 1993). Even these limited values may be useful for interpreting measurements made upon individual patients and more detailed distributions may be found in the original sources of the data. Note that if a subject's measurement is below the 5th percentile, appropriate for their age and sex, they are in the lowest 5% of the population, at the 50th centile they are exactly in the middle of the range and above the 95th percentile then they are in the top 5%.

WEIGHT

Body weight can be one of the most important and useful indicators of nutritional status, particularly if it is measured longitudinally (i.e. a series of measurements over time). Unintentional weight loss may be an important indicator of disease or of deteriorating nutritional status brought on by unsatisfactory socioeconomic conditions. Percentage weight loss over the preceding three months is one convenient way of quantifying this weight loss:

weight loss of up to 5%   –   mild depletion
weight loss 5–10%   –   moderate depletion
weight loss more than 10%   –   severe depletion

Oedema (excess tissue fluid) may disguise weight loss or it may be responsible for sudden increases in body weight. The presence of oedema should be noted and borne in mind when interpreting body weight measurements or changes. Oedema may, of itself, be an indicator of a nutritional or medical problem.

HEIGHT

Height is the simplest and most widely used measure of skeletal size. Cross sectional measures of heights in an adult population would be expected to show a decrease in average height with age. This would be partly due to a real decrease in height as people age but also due to the general trend for younger generations to be taller than their parents and grandparents. White *et al.* (1993) found just such a trend in a sample of English adults:

Mean height:	men 25–34 years	= 176.3 cm
	men 75+ years	= 168.5 cm
	women 25–34 years	= 163 cm
	women 75+ years	= 156 cm

BODY MASS INDEX

When both height and weight are measured the body mass index (BMI) can be calculated and used as a simple indicator of body fatness:

$$BMI = \frac{Body\ weight\ in\ kilograms}{(Height\ in\ metres)^2}$$

The following classification system for BMI is very widely used:

BMI less than 20	–	underweight
20–25	–	ideal range
25–30	–	overweight
30+	–	obese

A BMI of less than 19 in an older person would indicate the need for a more thorough assessment as there is an increased probability of the person being undernourished. A BMI of less than 16 would indicate that the subject is seriously undernourished.

The underlying assumption when using BMI to indicate body fatness is that differences in weight for any given height are largely due to differences in body fat content. Two age-related changes may make the use of the above standard classification system for BMI less reliable:

• loss of height with age
• an increase in the fat to lean ratio in older people.

Table 6.2 shows two sets of norms for BMI obtained from samples of elderly British people. The norms obtained from the 1993 publication are all substantially greater than those from the 1984 publication. These differences are consistent with other evidence from the population as a whole that average BMIs have risen in recent years and that there has been a large increase in the proportion of adults who are overweight or obese. These changes may reduce the sensitivity of single anthropometric measurements as indicators of unsatisfactory nutritional status since if people are overweight they will take longer to reach an anthropometric threshold taken to indicate malnutrition.

DEMI-SPAN AND KNEE HEIGHT

For their height to be measured the person must be able to stand erect with the eyes at right angles to the ground. This may not be possible for many elderly people and so alternative measures of skeletal size have been sought. Demi-span is one such measure; it is the distance from the web of the fingers (between the middle and ring fingers) and the sternal notch when the subject's arm is held horizontally to the side (with support if necessary); it is usually measured with a steel tape. COMA (1992) recommended that demi-span measurements should be included in all nutritional surveys of older people. It has been suggested that demi-span might decline less with age than does height and so any age-related changes in demi-span with age in cross sectional studies might be expected to be largely cohort effects (due to the changes in height between generations). The change in demi-span with age in the English cross sectional sample of White *et al.* (1993) was, in percentage terms, very similar to the decline in height noted above:

e.g. Mean demi-span

	men 25–34 years	= 83.0 cm
men 75+ years	= 79.6 cm
women 25–34 years	= 75.5 cm
women 75+ years	= 72.1 cm

White *et al.* (1993) derived the following equations for estimating height from demi-span measurements in people aged over 55 years:

(all measurements in centimetres)

$$\text{Height for men} = (1.2 \times \text{demi-span}) + 71$$

$$\text{Height for women} = (1.2 \times \text{demi-span}) + 67$$

This enables BMI to be estimated from measurements of weight and demi-span. Demi-span measurements can be also be used to derive indices with body weight which are analogous to the body mass index, two such indices are the mindex and the demiquet:

$$\text{Mindex} = \frac{\text{weight in kg}}{\text{demi-span in m}}$$

$$\text{Demiquet} = \frac{\text{weight in kg}}{(\text{demi-span in m})^2}$$

The changes in both mindex and demiquet with age are similar to those seen for BMI in Figure 4.1 (White *et al.*, 1993) and both mindex and demiquet correlated very highly with BMI. White *et al.* (1993) concluded that mindex was probably a better index of obesity than demiquet. Table 6.2 shows some norms for both mindex and demiquet. The Royal College of Nursing has published a set of nutrition standards for older people (RCN, 1993) and this contains a ready-reckoner that gives estimates of the BMI from measurements of demi-span and body weight. Knee height is measured in a seated position and is the height from the floor to the knee joint space. Both the shortness of the distance and the difficulty of precisely locating the knee joint space increases the relative size of measurement errors. The following equations can be used to estimate height from knee height:

$$\text{height for men} = 64.19 + (\text{knee height} \times 2.03) - (0.04 \times \text{age})$$

$$\text{height for women} = 84.88 + (\text{knee height} \times 1.83) - (0.24 \times \text{age})$$

(all measurements in centimetres)

UPPER ARM CIRCUMFERENCE

If patients cannot be weighed (for example if they cannot get out of bed) then the circumference of the mid part of the upper arm (mid-arm circumference, MAC) can be a useful alternative to weight as a measure of nutritional status. Single measurements may be difficult to interpret because of the absence of good standards but longitudinal changes can be a reasonably sensitive indicator of changes in body weight. A value of less than 22 cm may be considered to indicate increased risk of malnutrition.

Mid-arm muscle circumference (MAMC) has been quite widely used as a simple measure of lean body mass. The circumference of the mid upper arm is measured with a tape and then the triceps skinfold is measured with skinfold calipers and used as an indicator of the amount of subcutaneous fat in the area. MAMC is then calculated using the formula:

$$\text{MAMC} = \text{mid-arm circumference} - (\pi \times \text{triceps skinfold})$$

Once again, this can be particularly useful as a longitudinal indicator of changes in lean body mass over time.

Some norms for both MAC and MAMC are shown in Table 6.2. It should be borne in mind that these are British norms of ten years ago.

One other frequently used measure that is derived from the mid- arm muscle circumference is the arm muscle area. It is derived using the following equation:

$$\text{Arm muscle area} = \frac{(\text{mid-arm muscle circumference})^2}{4\pi}$$

SKINFOLD CALIPERS

The most widely used direct measure of fatness in people is measurement of skinfold thickness using skinfold calipers. These spring loaded calipers exert a constant pressure on a fold of skin; the thickness of the skinfold is indicated on a meter. The thickness of the skinfold will be largely dependent upon the amount of fat stored subcutaneously in the region of the skinfold. Skinfold thicknesses are measured at several sites and the assumption is made that the amount of fat stored subcutaneously at these sites (as measured by the skinfold thickness) will be representative of the total amount of body fat. Typically, skinfold thickness is determined at four sites:

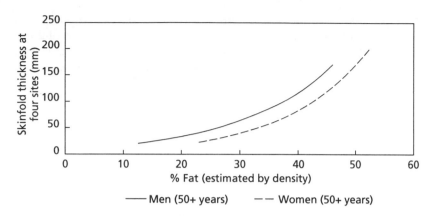

Figure 6.1 Relationship between skin fold thickness and body fatness in elderly adults. Data source: Durnin and Womersley (1974)

- over the triceps muscle
- over the biceps
- in the subscapular region
- in the supra iliac region.

The total of these four skinfolds is then translated into an estimate of percentage body fat using a calibration table or formula. Figure 6.1 shows the relationship between the sum of these four skinfolds and the estimated percentage body fat (estimated by body density) in men and women aged over 50 years.

The single triceps skinfold thickness is sometimes used in nutritional surveys – it has the obvious advantage in such circumstances that it can be measured quickly and without the need for subjects to undress. It can also be used as a quick guide to the level of fat stores in individual subjects. Some norms are shown in Table 6.2.

The apparent simplicity of these skinfold procedures should not obscure the fact that considerable skill and experience is required to get reliable results using them. According to COMA (1992), there are particular problems with the use of this method in older people which makes it useful only as a rough guide to their fatness, for example:

- there are age-related changes in the compressibility of the skinfold that have not yet been properly described
- there are age-related changes in the proportion of subcutaneous to deep body fat.

Biochemical assessment

Biochemical tests are generally the most sensitive indicators of nutritional status. They yield objective and quantitative results but have the disadvantage of being relatively labour intensive and expensive. They require laboratory facilities and trained personnel to perform the analysis and also often require trained personnel to take blood samples. Another problem of several biochemical tests is the lack of reliable and appropriate standards.

Where standards do exist they have usually been derived from studies with younger adults and there has seldom been direct testing of their suitability for use with elderly people. COMA (1992) highlighted the need for better biochemical indicators of vitamin C, zinc, copper and antioxidant status.

Serum albumin. This has been widely used an indicator of general nutritional status; a low serum albumin concentration may indicate energy/protein malnutrition. A number of other medical condition also result in reduced serum albumin (e.g. liver and renal diseases, some cancers and infections) and this would need to be borne in mind when interpreting low values. Albumin concentrations tend to fall slowly because albumin is degraded slowly and so this is not a good indicator of acute depletion but may indicate chronic undernutrition.

The following ranges may be useful guides when interpreting serum albumin measurements:

Nutritional status	Serum albumin g/litre
normal range	35–45
mild depletion	30–35
moderate depletion	25–30
severe depletion	< 25

Serum transferrin. Transferrin is the protein which transports iron in blood plasma. It is thought to be a more sensitive measure of current nutritional status than serum albumin as it falls more rapidly during undernutrition.

Again, some other conditions affect iron transport (e.g. chronic infection, trauma and liver disease) and thus may also affect the serum transferrin level.

The following ranges for serum transferrin may be a useful guide to interpreting values:

Nutritional status	Serum transferrin g/litre
normal range	2.5–3.0
mild depletion	1.5–2.5
moderate depletion	1.0–1.5
severe malnutrition	< 1.0

TESTS FOR SPECIFIC NUTRIENTS

Many of the biochemical measures of nutrient status involve measuring the level of the nutrient or one of its derivatives in blood plasma/serum or blood cells. Some examples of the biochemical indices of the status for particular nutrients are shown in Table 6.3 together with some guides as to the values that indicate satisfactory nutrient status.

Two of the tests noted in Table 6.3 are examples of enzyme activation tests. These activation tests rely on the fact that several of the B vitamins act as cofactors or coenzymes that are essential for the functioning of particular enzymes. In vitamin deficiency, the activity of the enzyme will be reduced because of lack of availability of the vitamin-derived cofactor. The method

Table 6.3 Selected biochemical indicators of nutrient status that may be used in the nutritional assessment of elderly people

Test/ marker	Nutrient	'Ideal' values
Serum albumin	energy/protein	35–45 g/l
Serum transferrin	energy/protein	2.5–3.0 g/l
Erythrocyte glutathione reductase activation	riboflavin	EGRAC <1.3
Erythrocyte transketolase activation	thiamin	ETKLAC <1.2
Plasma/serum pyridoxal phosphate	vitamin B_6	5–23 µg/l
Serum vitamin B_{12}	vitamin B_{12}	>130 ng/l
Serum folate Red cell folate	folate	>3 µg/l >150 µg/l
Plasma/serum vitamin C Leucocyte vitamin C	vitamin C	>2 mg/l >15 µg/10^8 cells
Plasma 25-hydroxy cholecalciferol (vit D)	vitamin D	>8 µg/l
Blood haemoglobin Serum ferritin	iron	>11.5 g/dl >25 µg/l
Serum/plasma zinc	zinc	10–18 µmol/l

involves measuring the activity of the enzyme in samples of red blood cells with and without the addition of excess of the cofactor. If the activity of the enzyme is greatly increased by addition of the cofactor, this indicates that lack of the cofactor was limiting enzyme activity and thus that the donor of the cells had some deficiency of the vitamin. For example, glutathione reductase is an enzyme present in red blood cells whose activity is dependent upon the presence of a cofactor that is derived from riboflavin; the enzyme cannot function in the absence of the cofactor. In riboflavin deficiency, the activity of this enzyme is low because of reduced availability of the cofactor. To perform the activation test, the activity of glutathione reductase is measured in two samples of red cells from the subject – one has had excess of the riboflavin-derived cofactor added whilst the other has not. The ratio of these two activities – the erythrocyte glutathione reductase activation coefficient (EGRAC) – is a measure of the subject's dietary riboflavin status. An EGRAC of less than 1.3 is taken to indicate satisfactory riboflavin status.

It would be fair to say that many of the methods listed in Table 6.3 are more often used as research tools or for confirmation of a clinical diagnosis than for screening individuals. They would be used, for example, by those doing in-depth surveys of the nutritional status of groups or populations of elderly people.

Table 6.4 Some advantages and disadvantages of prospective and retrospective methods of measuring food intake

All methods:
• rely upon the honesty of the subjects
• assume that the monitored period is representative of the subject's habitual intake
• rely upon printed food tables or a computer database in order to translate food portions into energy and nutrient intakes (use of food tables critically reviewed in Webb, 1995).
Retrospective methods
quick and cheap
require little commitment from the subjects
participation rates are high
subjects cannot change their eating behaviour in response to monitoring
BUT
very subject to memory errors
retrospective quantification of food portions is difficult
interviewer may influence subjects
Prospective methods
less prone to memory and quantification errors
BUT
require commitment and competent record keeping by subjects
subjects may modify behaviour in response to monitoring, e.g. to impress investigator, to simplify record keeping or simply because their awareness has been heightened by the recording process

Dietary assessment

There is a range of methods available for estimating the food and nutrient intakes of individuals. Investigators are usually seeking a reliable measure of the habitual intake of the subject but all of the methods are subject to considerable errors and uncertainties. The methods may be retrospective, relying upon the subject's recall of what they have eaten in the past, or prospective, a planned recording of consumption as it occurs. The choice of method will be dependent upon several factors such as:

• the purpose of the measurement
• the competence and commitment of the subjects
• the time and resources available to the investigators.

Some of the advantages and disadvantages of prospective and retrospective methods are listed in Table 6.4.

RECALL METHOD

The subject is asked to recall all of the food and fluid consumed over a period of time, usually the previous 24 hours (24 hour recall). This provides information on 'yesterday's' intake but of course that may not be typical of their

Table 6.5 Some examples of probe questions for a 24 hour recall

Breakfast
At what time did you eat breakfast today? Say, 8 a.m. reply.
What did you have for breakfast today?
If reply is toast:
How many slices of bread?
What type of bread/size of loaf?
What did you put on the bread?
How much?
Can you describe how much – about one teaspoon or two?
Did you have anything to drink?
If reply is tea:
Cup or mug? What size? How many?
What did you put in the tea? – sugar, honey, milk? How much?
Morning snacks and drinks
When did you last eat or drink anything? Say 11 a.m. reply.
Did you eat anything between 8 a.m. (breakfast) and 11 a.m.?
If reply – yes
What was that?
A biscuit.
How many? What type? Anything to drink?
Yes, tea – follow up questions as for breakfast above.
What did you have at 11 a.m.? Follow up questions as above.

habitual intake. The interviewer tries to get the subject to give as complete a record as possible; snacks and drinks are particularly likely to be forgotten. Some illustrative examples of probe questions are shown in Table 6.5. This is likely to be the starting point for any dietary assessment of an individual by a dietitian and is also likely to be used when designing a therapeutic diet for an individual. Modifying existing dietary practices, as identified by dietary recall methods, is likely to produce greater compliance with therapeutic diets than simply trying to impose a standard dietary prescription.

The following hints may be useful in improving the reliability and validity of recall assessments.

- It is generally best to ask about times of day as the meaning of some meal titles (like 'tea' or 'dinner') varies.
- Interviewers must try not to make assumptions about other people's food combinations based upon their own practices.
- Use of cues, like 'Who was around at the time?' may assist people with recall.
- It is important to quantify portion sizes and the size of cups and plates used. Sometimes food models are used to assist people in quantifying portion sizes. If a meal is shared, the proportion eaten by the subject needs to be determined.
- The interviewer must avoid giving any indications of approval, disapproval or surprise at clients responses, otherwise the responses of the client may well be biased by these interviewer reactions.
- If prepared dishes are eaten then some estimation of the recipe is helpful. For commercially prepared products the brand should be ascertained.
- It may be possible to cross-check some items by some general questions at the end of the interview. For example, are daily milk purchases consistent with the milk consumption in the record? can inconsistencies be accounted for by wastage or by giving milk to a cat?

DIET HISTORY

This involves more detailed questioning and attempts to identify what the client normally eats and drinks. A typical meal pattern is identified with details of quantities usually consumed and usual preparation methods. Any recent changes in food and fluid intake are identified, together with the subject's explanation of why have they occurred.

FOOD FREQUENCY

This involves asking subjects how often they eat particular foods e.g. daily, weekly, rarely, never. This technique can be useful when assessing the intake of particular nutrients. For example questions about the frequency of consumption of fruits, vegetables and juices or fortified cordials may give an indication of the subject's habitual intake of vitamin C.

Some food frequency checklists have been developed which have a scoring system that seeks to screen for particular nutritional problems. Figure 6.2 shows an example of one of these screening tools, the NAGE checklist. The

Name _____ Completed by _____

Address _____ _____

_____ Date _____

General Questions.
1. Do you usually eat   Breakfast   yes/no
                      Mid-day lunch/dinner   yes/no
                      Tea/evening meal   yes/no
2. Have you lost or gained more than 1 stone
    in weight in the last year, without trying to?
                      Gained weight   yes/no
                      Lost weight   yes/no
3. Are you on a special diet?   yes/no
    (eg diabetic, high fibre, reducing)   Type _____
4. Are you taking any food/drink supplements ?   yes/no
    (eg Complan, Bengers, Build Up).
    If yes, what?   _____
5. Are you taking any laxatives, vitamin supplements
    cod liver oil, iron tablets etc.?   yes/no
    If yes, what?   _____
Please consider the answers to questions 1–5 when using the checklist as they will influence your advice and action.

NOTE. As you ask the questions in sections 1–4, circle the score for each answer. If twice as much is eaten *double the score* and if eaten less often than once a week or never, *score zero [0]*. If the score is *under 10 in any section* please consult the relevant information in the guidance notes.

Section 1 **IRON**   Total _____

How often do you eat?	weekly	alt.days	daily
Black pudding.	4	10	20
Liver, kidney, heart.	3	6	12
Liver pate/sausage/faggots.	2	4	8
Red meat, corned beef.	2	4	8
Egg.	1	2	4
Breakfast cereal.	1	2	4
Wholemeal bread – 3 slices.	0	1	3
Dark green vegetables.	0	1	3
Pulse vegetables eg. lentils.	0	1	3

Section 2 **VITAMIN C**   Total _____

How often do you eat?	weekly	alt.days	daily
Citrus fruit eg. orange.	2	5	10
Soft fruit eg. strawberries, blackcurrants. (not tinned).	2	5	10
Grapefruit/orange/tomato juice (not tinned).	1	3	6
Vit C enriched cordial eg. blackcurrant.	1	3	6
Potatoes incl. instant.	1	3	6
Green vege/tomato/salad.	1	2	3
Banana/tinned mandarin.	1	2	3

Section 3 **CALCIUM/VITAMIN D**   Total _____

How often do you eat?	weekly	alt.days	daily
1/2 pint milk (drinks/cereal).	1	3	6
Sardines/pilchards.	2	4	8
Cheese (1 oz).	1	2	4
Yoghurt/ice cream.	1	2	3
Milk pudding/custard/evap.	1	2	3

Remember the best way to get vitamin D is by going out into the sunshine. Housebound people are particularly at risk of deficiency.

Section 4 **FIBRE**   Total _____

How often do you eat?	weekly	alt.days	daily
Wholegrain breakfast cereals.	3	4	5
Wholemeal bread/roll (3 slice).	2	3	4
Wholegrain biscuits /crackers/crispbread (3–6).	1	2	3
Pulses include baked beans.	1	2	3
Fruit.	0	1	2
Vegetables/salad.	0	1	2
White bread.	0	0	1
Chapatti/rice/pasta.	0	0	1

It is important to drink at least 8 cups of fluid a day to prevent constipation.

Figure 6.2 The nutrition assessment checklist. Developed by: Nutrition Advisory Group of the British Dietetic Association for Elderly People

Table 6.6 A sample page from a completed food diary

Time	Description of food or drink	Amount of serving, e.g. cup, slice, spoonful	Leftover
07:30	Weetabix semi-skimmed milk sugar coffee with semi-skimmed milk, no sugar wholemeal toast butter marmalade	2 biscuits 1 cup 1 teaspoon 2 cups 2 medium slices large/medium loaf medium layers 2 teaspoons	
10:30	coffee with whole milk, no sugar chocolate digestive biscuits	1 mug 2	
12:30	wholemeal bread butter ham tomato cucumber banana apple	3 slices large loaf thinly spread 3 thin slices 1 medium 6 slices 1 medium 1 medium	
15:30	tea with whole milk, no sugar	1 mug	
17:30	coffee with semi-skimmed milk	1 mug	
18:30	chicken breast (fried in olive oil with skin, no bone) jacket potato butter baked beans orange dry white wine coffee with semi-skimmed milk, no sugar	1 1 large 1 teaspoon 2 tablespoons 1 large 2 glasses 2 cups	
20:00	unsweetened orange juice	1 glass	
21:00	lager beer	1 large can	
23:00	drinking chocolate (made with semi-skimmed milk)	1 mug	

Nutrition Advisory Group for Elderly People (NAGE) is a group of dietitians within the British Dietetic Association who have particular interests in the nutrition of the elderly. This checklist was designed as a screening tool to be used by Community Care workers to help them to identify nutritional problems amongst their clients. The checklist has an introductory section and then four sections each related to a specific nutritional problem. The general questions are designed to alert the worker to the potential for general malnutrition whereas the subsequent sections relate to four nutritional problems that are common amongst elderly people: anaemia, osteomalacia, vitamin C deficiency and constipation.

The checklist would be used in conjunction with some guidance notes. Thus, for example, if a client reports unintentional and significant weight loss then a medical referral to identify the cause would be the recommended response. The checklist, and others like it, serve not only their direct purpose of screening for specific nutritional problems but they also put food onto the agenda of the care workers; they heighten awareness of food and nutrition and highlight the importance of adequate food intake to maintaining or restoring health and wellbeing.

FOOD DIARY

The subject keeps a record in a diary of all the food and drink consumed over a specified period, often seven days. The subjects will need some instruction before undertaking the recording and the accuracy is improved if an experienced person checks the diary with the subject in order to clarify any ambiguities or correct obvious errors. A typical page from a completed food diary is shown in Table 6.6; note that this is an idealised record and it would probably require editing and clarification by a trained interviewer to obtain such a complete record with untrained subjects.

WEIGHED INVENTORY

This method is essentially a food diary in which the subject weighs all of the food consumed over the study period. It is the most time-consuming of all the methods and requires highly motivated subjects who are capable of accurately weighing and recording everything they consume. This method would most likely be used as a research or surveillance tool rather than as a diagnostic method of nutritional assessment. The major UK nutritional surveys (e.g. Gregory et al., 1990) have used this method.

Nutritional assessment in hospitals and residential homes

In Chapter 5, several sources were quoted that had found that elderly people may be offered amounts of food that do not supply their estimated needs for energy and nutrients. Therefore, the first question that needs to be addressed is 'do the meals provide adequate amounts of energy and nutrients?'. It is a relatively simple matter to roughly estimate the nutrient content of a daily menu if the portion sizes are given. If the proposed menu is inadequate in energy and/or nutrients, portion sizes can be adjusted to compensate. Such calculations need not be restricted to institutional meals; similar principles can be applied to any meals provided for elderly people (e.g. meals at luncheon clubs, day centres and meals on wheels). It would seem reasonable to expect that any main meal provided by these routes should contain at least one-third of the daily nutrient needs of an elderly person. Allowance needs to be made for likely nutrient losses, particularly losses of water soluble vitamins in the period between preparation and consumption. These losses may be substantial if the food is kept warm for extended periods prior to serving.

Of course, ensuring that the meals provided are nutritionally adequate is only a first step. Several meal-related factors and client-related factors will determine what proportion of the proffered food is actually consumed. The acceptability and palatability of the food will affect nutrient intakes and this needs to be actively monitored.

Some hospitals have developed computerised databases which contain the nutrient contents of standard portions of all the menu items supplied by the hospital kitchens (plus common items supplied by visitors or bought by patients). This provides an opportunity for relatively easy monitoring of nutritional intakes of selected patients. The meals offered to the patient are recorded together with the proportion of the food that remains uneaten at the end of each meal. This can then be keyed into the computer to give a reasonably accurate indication of the patients nutrient intake.

Medical screening of elderly people in the UK

Since April 1990 general practitioners working within the UK National Health Service have had a contractual obligation to carry out annual assessments of all patients over 75 years on their patient registers. This new obligation for screening of the elderly reflects the increasing priority attached to preventative medicine by the UK government. The hope is that this screening process will pick up previously unidentified needs and problems of older people, give an early warning of some impending problems, and allow the practitioner to review long-standing repeat prescriptions for drugs. The optimistic view of this screening procedure is that:

- it will improve the quality of life of many elderly people and 'add life to years' by allowing unrecognised problems to be dealt with at an earlier stage
- by identifying and intervening to ameliorate problems or potential problems at an early stage some later costs may be reduced (e.g. by reducing the number of random patient consultations or by providing community services that enable the elderly to remain independent for longer before their inability to cope results in their requiring institutional care)
- it may result in more efficient use of the budget for prescribed drugs by highlighting unnecessary and ineffective repeat prescriptions.

This screening initiative has itself also been criticised on several grounds including the following.

- That this extra domiciliary consultation for all over 75s adds substantially and unnecessarily to the workload of general practitioners – to quote Freer (1990), 'most older people are reasonably well and healthy and content, so that imposing universal domiciliary screening on an annual basis seems to be a wasteful use of limited resources, and to be inconsistent with the principle of targeted support to those in greatest need.' In practice, about 90% of people in this age group see their family doctor at least once a year and the average is six consultations per year. Much of the screening assessment work can thus be completed opportunistically during one of these surgery consultations. Only a small proportion of the over 75s (around 10%) would need to be contacted and offered an extra domiciliary visit. There is also no obligation for the doctor to actually carry out the screening procedure and it can be done by nurses attached to a general practice.
- The screening procedure may not identify new needs and problems but simply re-reveal common problems that are already well known to the doctor. It is also suggested that many of these chronic problems are incurable or that effective intervention is not possible because of lack of resources. If a screening procedure identifies some unmet social, economic, or medical needs of the patient then this is of little value if effective intervention is not possible because of resource limitations.

The assessment is under six headings – sensory function, mobility, mental state, physical condition, social environment and use of medicines. There are no guidelines as to what these actually mean so there has been a great variation in the way the initiative has been implemented across the UK.

This screening process is bound to highlight many common problems with a long history for the patient but it also provides an opportunity to identify less common and relatively new conditions in the individual client. Undernutrition and diabetes are clearly nutrition-related problems that may be first recognised by general screening and ameliorated by nutrition interventions. Impaired mobility and the social environment can affect the food consumed and the availability of the food, and hence affect the nutritional status of a particular individual.

Many screening tools are being developed to meet the needs of this programme and Freer (1990) suggests that these should concentrate on functional assessment rather than disease detection. For example, he suggests that in the field of mobility assessment, one should be screening for the ability to perform tasks like walking and climbing stairs rather than seeking to identify clinical problems that may affect mobility, like osteoarthritis. This should simplify the screening process and identify those patients who clearly have unmet needs. Once a functional problem has been identified then the cause can be sought and hopefully effective interventions made. Freer gives as an example, some very simple questions that can be used as the basis of a functional assessment of mental condition:

What is today's date?
What year is it?
What day of the week is it?

How old are you?
What is your date of birth?
What is your address?
What are the dates of World War I?
Who is the prime minister/monarch?
Can you count backwards from 20?

Three or more incorrect answers might indicate some mental deterioration and the number of extra errors might be a guide to the severity of the problem.

Examples of functional criteria that could be used for assessment under the six assessment headings are given below:

- **Sensory functions,** e.g. sight and hearing. Functional assessments here could include: problems with conversation or listening to the radio and television, ability to recognise faces across the room, ability to read a newspaper.
- **Mobility** Functional criteria here could be: the ability to walk unaided, ability to climb stairs, ability to rise unaided from a chair, ability to use public transport – getting on and off buses.
- **Mental condition** Criteria here could be: evidence of depression, altered sleeping patterns, alcohol abuse, memory loss or symptoms of dementia.
- **Physical condition** This includes such things as continence and the ability to cope with the everyday tasks of daily life. Functional assessment here could include: evidence of incontinence, laxative use, symptoms of prostate problems, polyuria, ability to prepare meals, ability to wash and dress unaided.
- **Social environment** Functional assessment here could include: frequency of social contact, receipt of all benefits to which they are entitled, suitability of heating systems and economic means to use them, adequate means of obtaining and preparing a varied and palatable diet.
- **The use of medicine** A review of medication to include both self-medication and prescribed medicines.

It is probably too early to make conclusive judgements on the effectiveness or otherwise of this screening initiative but in a short referenced article, Thompson (1993) has suggested that evidence of a beneficial impact of this screening is starting to emerge. In his own practice, Thompson reports that random consultations by elderly patients were almost halved in the year after he introduced screening and that his review of repeat prescriptions and compliance led to substantial savings on the drugs budget. He also quotes the results of several other studies that suggest that screening does identify a variety of previously unrecorded problems.

Nutritional screening

Screening in the community

The general screening of the over 75s in the UK described above provides an opportunity to include a nutritional assessment if simple, appropriate and valid nutritional screening tools are available and if there is heightened awareness amongst doctors, nurses and other health workers of the importance of good nutrition to the health and wellbeing of older people. The NAGE check-list (Figure 6.2) could for example be used to identify those patients whose dietary habits increase their risk from the specific nutritional problems that it is designed to identify. This checklist was designed to be used by non-specialists and comes with a set of guidance notes that explain its use, how to respond to particular problems highlighted by responses, and where to obtain further advice or guidance.

MINI NUTRITIONAL ASSESSMENT

Guigoz *et al.* (1994) have developed and validated a mini nutritional assessment that they suggest is suitable for use with frail elderly people be they in their own homes, residential accommodation or in hospital. They suggest that their assessment should be able to be completed in less than 15 minutes by a non-specialist assessor. The assessment consists of 18 questions arranged under four headings and there is a designated score for the available answers for each question. Clients would be classified as 'well-nourished', 'at risk' or 'malnourished' on the basis of their total score.

The four areas for the assessment questions are listed below.

Anthropometric assessment – four simple anthropometric measures of nutritional status are used:

- body mass index
- mid-arm circumference
- calf circumference
- weight loss in the preceding three months.

Global evaluation – this consists of six questions relating to:

- whether the client lives independently or not
- takes three or more prescription medicines daily
- has suffered from psychological stress or acute disease in the preceding three months
- their degree of mobility
- the presence or absence of neuropsychological problems
- the presence of pressure sores or skin ulcers.

Dietetic assessment – comprises six questions relating to:

- the number of full daily meals consumed
- consumption of specified minimum numbers of portions from the meat and milk food groups
- consumption of specified minimum numbers of portions of fruits and vegetables
- any recent loss of appetite, digestive problems or chewing/swallowing problems
- consumption of adequate daily amounts of fluids
- the client's degree of independence in feeding.

Subjective assessment – two questions that ask how the client views their own health and nutrition:

- whether they consider they have any nutritional problems
- how they view their health in comparison to that of other people of their own age.

RISK AND WARNING GRID

Davies and Knutson (1991) have developed a grid system designed to help identify those people who are at risk of malnutrition in the community (Figure 6.3). It is an initial assessment tool for nutrition that can be used in the community by people with very limited training related to nutrition but who are willing to look and report.

Along the horizontal axis are risk factors – these are major identifiable biological or environmental circumstances or events that increase the risk of malnutrition and therefore suggest the need for special care and attention. For example, being housebound is recognised as a risk factor, as is living alone, chronic bronchitis, poor dentition or no regular cooked meals. This does not mean that everybody who is housebound is malnourished, but it means as a risk factor it has the potential of contributing towards malnutrition.

Along the vertical axis are warning signals. Warning signals are observable circumstances that if left unchecked, might directly cause an 'at risk' individual to become malnourished. Warning signals could include: recent unintentional

Figure 6.3 The nutritional assessment grid.
Source: Davies and Knutson (1991)

WARNING SIGNALS (RISK FACTORS →)	Living alone	Housebound	No regular cooked meals	Low mental test score	Clinical diagnosis depression	Chronic bronchitis/emphysema	Gastrectomy	Poor dentition and/or difficulty in swallowing
Recent unintended weight change + or – 3 kg (7 lb)	•	•	•	•	•	•	•	•
Physical disability affecting food shopping, preparation or intake	•	•	•		•	•		
Lack of sunlight		•			•			
Bereavement and/or observed depression/loneliness	•	•	•	•	•	•		
Mental confusion affecting eating	•		•	•				
High alcohol consumption	•		•		•			
Polypharmacy/long-term medication	•		•	•	•			
Missed meals/snacks/fluids	•	•	•	•	•	•	•	•
Food wastage/rejection	•	•	•	•	•	•	•	•
Insufficient food stores at home	•	•	•	•	•	•		
Lack of fruit/juices/vegetables	•	•	•					•
Low budget for food	•		•					
Poor nutritional knowledge		•	•	•				

weight change, bereavement, high alcohol consumption, missed meals or insufficient food stores at home. Those warning signals that apply to any particular risk factor are indicated by a bullet at the appropriate point on the grid. When using the grid, the first step is to mark any risk factors that apply to the client – the presence of four or more risk factors would suggest that the client was at high risk. Once the risk factors have been noted one would look for those warning signals appropriate for these risk factors and circle them in the grid.

The warning signals are likely to be cumulative and so the presence of several warning signals for any risk factor would increase the chances that this risk factor was leading to malnutrition. For example, food wastage could simply be an example of an unpopular meal, but if found in conjunction with depression, high alcohol consumption and recent weight loss this would make the probability that there was a nutritional problem much greater than just the random observation of an uneaten meal.

DAVIES AND SCOTTS' CARE AND ASSISTANCE GRID

The current policy of the UK government is to encourage 'Care in the Community'. The general aim is to reduce the number of people in residential care; this applies not just to the elderly but across the whole spectrum of care (e.g. the mentally ill and those with physical and mental disabilities). In theory, services and resources should be made available to enable the elderly to compensate for their declining capabilities and to ameliorate their impact so that they can continue to live independent or semi-independent lives for longer. Services such as meals on wheels, home helps to assist with domestic chores, mobility allowances, sheltered accommodation, where a warden is on hand for help when required, etc. Institutional care is increasingly being seen as a last resort reserved for those so severely handicapped by illness or disability that they are completely incapable of functioning independently.

As the number of elderly people living within the community grows, so the demand for community meals and other services also seems certain to continue growing. Davies and Scotts (1994) have designed a grid that is intended to help identify those in need of some assistance and the nature and level of assistance that is required and acceptable to the client, and also to identify the need for development of services in particular areas. On the horizontal axis of the grid is the range of community services that could be offered. Davies and Scotts (1994) suggest 15 service provisions and 17 'enabling services' that could be included in this list.

Provided services would include:

- meals on wheels
- a home help bringing meals from a freezer in sheltered accommodation
- various types of residential care
- lunch clubs
- mini freezer projects (provision of a small freezer and cooker and a month's supply of frozen meals)
- visits by a member of the primary care team.

'**Enabling services**' are those that require little or no input of resources from the local authority but may supplement or replace provided services. Some examples would be:

- a pensioner's meals provided by local pubs and restaurants
- food and drink delivered by a milkman
- deliveries by local retailers
- excursions to shops or transport to a lunch club by a neighbour or volunteer
- deliveries of frozen meals by a manufacturer.

On the vertical axis of the grid is a list of up to 33 risk factors and warning signals for malnutrition similar to those seen earlier in Davies and Knutson's risk assessment grid (Figure 6.3). For each of the risk factors/warning signals certain 'provided' or 'enabling' services are asterisked as appropriate for that particular situation. When assessing the needs of a client, the risk factors/warning signals would be identified and the appropriate interventions highlighted. The choice of service provided would then be made on the basis of acceptability to the client and the local availability of services. Use of this grid could also identify the need for provision of new local services; this could be particularly useful if relatively cheap enabling or provided services can be identified that might reduce the need for more expensive provided services.

This grid is intended to increase efficiency in the use of finite local resources and make sure that resources are directed towards those who need them most and those who will accept them. By identifying the cheapest services that are appropriate and acceptable to the client the benefits obtained from finite resources can be maximised.

Complete in first week _____ Date: _____		
Name: _____ Ward: _____ Age: _____		
Weight _____ Height: (Arm span height if not known) _____ BMI: (see chart)_____		
Change in weight:	Last six months _____	Last month: _____
BUILD/WEIGHT FOR HEIGHT	**SEX**	**SOCIAL FACTORS (you may code more than one)**
Overweight (visual) 2 Average (visual) 0 Below average (visual) 2 Very thin (visual) 4 OR BMI over 30 2 BMI 19–24 0 BMI 16–18 2 BMI less than 16 4 PLUS weight loss 10% in 6 months 4 (i.e. 6 kg loss from 60 kg) 5% in one month 5 (i.e. 3 kg loss from 60 kg)	Female 1 Male 2 **FOOD CONSUMPTION (you may code more than one)** All food and drink taken 0 3/4 food and drink taken 1 1/2 food and drink taken 2 1/4 food and drink taken 3 No food taken; takes drinks 4 No food or drink taken 5 *Additional factors:* Chewing difficulties 3 Swallowing difficulties 5 Pureed diet 4 Other special diet 3	Independent 0 Dependent on family/carers for meals 1 Dependent on others for meals 3 Difficulties in food preparation 2 Housebound 2 Lives alone 3 Recently bereaved 4 **ADDITIONAL FACTORS (you may code more than one)** Pain 3:4 Infection/repeated chest infections/UTI infections* 3:4 Pressure sores 4 Drugs (4 or more regularly) 3 Major surgery recently 4 Emergency fracture of femur 4 GI tract disease/diarrhoea 4 CVA 4 Breathlessness 4 Constipation/impaction 3:4
'EYEBALL' TEST (you may code more than one)	**MOOD (you may code more than one)**	
Healthy skin 0 Dry skin 1 Dehydrated 2 Poor colour 3 Evidence of weight loss – look at arms, legs & buttocks 4	Alert/interested 0 Apathetic 1 Anorexia/food refusal 3:4 Mild to moderate confusion 3 Severe dementia 4	
SCORE: Less than 10: OK	**10–19: Mod Risk 20–29: High Risk**	**30 + Very High Risk**

Figure 6.4 An example of a nutritional screening tool designed for use with elderly hospital patients. Reproduced from RCN (1993) courtesy of Meta Greenfield, Lifespan Healthcare, Cambridge

Screening in hospitals

Many patients, both young and old, who enter hospital are malnourished on admission and in a majority of patients weight loss and a deterioration in nutritional status occurs during their stay (KFC, 1992, McWhirter and Pennington, 1994). As a result of the increased awareness of this problem, a number of screening tools have been developed to assess rapidly the nutritional status of hospital patients at admission and to monitor any deterioration in nutritional status whilst in hospital. In 1993 a working party set up by the Royal College of Nursing produced a report entitled *Nutrition standards for the older adult* which focused upon the nurse's role in feeding older adults (RCN, 1993). As a parallel development, the dietetic profession produced *Standards of care for the dietitian working with the older adult in hospital* (NAGE 1993). One particular standard focuses on nutrition screening of the individual. It states 'the dietitian sets up a screening system with other professional staff whereby patients admitted to hospital are screened to identify those at risk nutritionally.' The expected outcome is that all patient nutritional needs will be identified and recorded as part of the nursing care plan. At risk patients and those requiring advice on therapeutic diets will be referred to the dietitian.

Most questionnaires aimed at nutritional screening of hospital patients include questions about some or all of the following:

- current food intake
- recent weight changes
- appetite
- swallowing or chewing difficulties and mouth condition
- medical and physical condition
- mental state
- socioeconomic circumstances.

Figure 6.4 shows an example of one of these screening tools that has been designed specifically for older patients.

Screening of residential homes

Just as the social and economic environment may have a profound influence upon the prevalence of malnutrition in the community, so institution-related factors may affect the nutritional wellbeing of the elderly resident in residential homes for the elderly. Davies and Holdsworth (1979) identified 26 potential risk factors that they thought might contribute to malnutrition in residential homes. They incorporated these risk factors into an A–Z checklist for assessing residential homes. In their original development and validation of the checklist, a pair of experienced investigators administered questionnaires to the head of the home, the cook and the residents, and there was also a list of questions about the home that were filled in by the investigators themselves. These questionnaire responses were used to grade each one of the risk factors as high, medium or low. When people know that they are being assessed by some external group then putting the questions on the checklist directly to the head of the home is unlikely to produce reliable responses and an objective assessment. Under these circumstances the investigators must use the questionnaire and their own observations made during an extended visit to arrive at their judgement for each item on the checklist. The completed checklist can then be used to compare homes and also to highlight particular problems with a view to suggesting improvements. The checklist can also be useful as a self-assessment tool for those running residential homes and seeking to identify weaknesses in their own practices with a view to raising their own standards. The checklist is reproduced in Figure 6.5 in a format appropriate for self-assessment by the managers of residential homes.

Every home has its risk factors. Pick out those which apply to your establishment and ask yourself: Why does it occur? Is it a 'high', 'moderate' or 'low' risk to the residents? What steps can be taken to lessen the risk?

A. Weekly cyclic menus or monotony of menu.
B. Difficulties with tea/supper meal menus.
C. Tea/supper meal on or before 5 p.m.
D. Lack of rapport between head of home and cook, or cook resists or resents suggestions.
E. Residents' suggestions (e.g. for recipes) unheeded. Residents' need for special diets ignored. Inadequate committee contact.
F. Residents not allowed choice of portion size or poor portion control or no second helpings available.
G. No heed taken of food wastage.
H. Very little home-style cooking.
I. No special occasion for food treats from local community or from the Home, apart from Christmas dinner.
J. For active residents: poor or no facilities for independence in providing food and drink e.g. tea making.
K. Hot foods served lukewarm or poor flavouring.
L. Poor presentation of food – including table setting, appearance of dining room.
M. Unfriendly or undignified waitress service. Meal too rushed.
N. No observation of weight changes of the residents.
O. No help in feeding very frail residents. No measures taken to protect other residents from offensive eating habits.
P. Head of Home and cook lacking basic nutritional or catering knowledge. Isolation from possible help.
Q. Lengthy period between preparation, cooking and serving. Time lag between staff meals and resident meals, especially affecting vegetables.
R. Lack of vitamin C foods or risk of unnecessary destruction of vitamin C.
S. Few vitamin D foods used, combined with lack of exposure to sunlight.
T. Low fibre diet and complaints of constipation.
U. Possible low intake of other nutrients – e.g. iron, folate and B_{12}.
V. Preponderance of convenience food of poor nutritional content.
W. Disproportionate costs between:
        i) animal protein
        ii) fruit and vegetables
        iii) energy foods.
X. Obvious food perks to staff to detriment of residents' meals. High proportion of food served to others.
Y. Conditions conducive to food poisoning. Lack of cleanliness.
Z. Recommendations may not be implemented.

Figure 6.5 A–Z checklist of potential nutritional risk factors in residential homes.
Source: Davies and Holdsworth (1979)

Improving the nutritional status of elderly people in residential homes and the community

Aims and scope of the chapter

In this chapter, we have sought to identify ways in which the nutritional status of elderly people might be improved. The chapter begins with a brief discussion of the impact of undernutrition upon the health of the elderly community and the likely benefits of improved nutritional support. There then follows a brief discussion of some of the general measures and changes that might improve the nutritional status of the elderly.

We have considered the quality of some specific service provisions, namely the availability and quality of community meals and the quality of catering in residential and nursing homes.

Finally, we have tried to identify ways of reducing the risks of food poisoning when catering for the elderly.

Impact of malnutrition in the community

There have been numerous studies that have looked at the impact of malnutrition in hospital patients and some of the ways in which malnutrition hinders recovery from illness, increases rates of complications during illness, and generally increases the costs of care (overviewed in KFC, 1992 and discussed more fully in Chapter 5).

Undernutrition and starvation also lead to a variety of adverse changes in healthy people (brief referenced review in KFC, 1992). For example, undernourishment leads to:

- reduced psychological wellbeing (increased anxiety, depression, apathy and loss of concentration)
- depressed immune function (Chandra, 1993)
- reduced muscle function (reduced strength and increased susceptibility to fatigue)
- loss of cardiac muscle and reduced cardiac function
- wasting of respiratory muscles and reduced respiratory response to oxygen deficit
- increased risk of hypothermia, particularly in elderly patients and this may increase incapacity and the risk of falls and injury.

Changes such as these would be expected to increase the general risk of illness and injury amongst the elderly so that undernutrition may be a cause of illness and injury as well as being a consequence of illness and an exacerbating influence upon existing illness and injury. Some general support for this proposition is provided by the predictive relationship between low anthropometric indices of nutritional status and subsequent mortality amongst the general elderly population (e.g. Mattila *et al.*, 1986; Campbell *et al.*, 1990; Exton-Smith, 1988).

Mowe *et al.* (1994) provide some more direct evidence that undernutrition may be a significant cause of illness in the elderly. They made a detailed nutritional assessment of a large sample of elderly patients (70+ years) admitted to an Oslo hospital because of an acute illness (e.g. stroke, myocardial infarction, pneumonia). They also assessed the nutritional status of a large, matched sample of elderly people living at home within the catchment area of this hospital. They confirmed several earlier reports that undernutrition is often present in elderly people at the time of their admission to hospital (in their study 50–60% of admissions were undernourished). The nutritional status of the hospital group was much worse than that of the home group using a battery of measures of nutritional status; 86% of the home subjects showed no sign of malnutrition compared to only 43% of the hospital group. They found that poor food intake in the month prior to admission was much more common in the hospital group than the home group:

- two-thirds of the hospital group reported inadequate energy intakes in the month before admission compared to one-third of the home group
- many more of the hospital group had intakes of vitamins and trace elements below 66% of the US RDA

- prevalence of problems with buying and preparing foods was greater in the hospital group
- eating difficulties were more prevalent in the hospital group
- members of the hospital group were more likely to have reported a reduced enjoyment from eating in the period prior to admission.

They suggested that reduced energy and nutrient intakes in the period prior to admission leads to reduced nutritional status and that this may be causally linked to increased risk of admission to hospital.

One would need to be cautious about concluding from studies such as those above that undernutrition is a major cause of non-nutritional illness and injury in the elderly even though there is overwhelming evidence that undernutrition and illness are associated. Very elderly people tend to lose weight in their final years, and so perhaps declining body weight is one of the indicators of physiological ageing that will inevitably predict mortality risk (see Chapter 4). Some undernutrition amongst the elderly is inevitably the result of chronic illness and disability and the presence of these problems is also likely to increase the risk of acute illnesses requiring hospital admission. Thus studies like those of Campbell et al. (1990) and Mowe et al. (1994) might tend to overstate the role of malnutrition as a major and primary cause of illness amongst the elderly.

Conclusion

There is little doubt that malnutrition has a major exacerbating effect upon illness and injury amongst all age groups. Illness is also more prevalent amongst poorly nourished populations. Almost certainly, undernutrition plays some role in precipitating illness and injury amongst elderly people although it is difficult to quantify its relative importance as a primary cause of non-nutritional illnesses and injuries.

Classification of malnutrition in the elderly

Davies (1988) has suggested that malnutrition in the elderly may be divided into four broad categories, as follows.

- **Specific:** a particular nutrient deficiency or nutrition-related disease such as scurvy, pellagra or osteomalacia.
- **Longstanding:** a long period of inadequate eating leading to clinical micronutrient and/or energy-protein deficiencies.
- **Sudden:** an acute medical problem or social disturbance (e.g. bereavement or admission to a residential home) that triggers marked changes in food intake and precipitates malnutrition.
- **Recurrent:** in an older person whose baseline intakes and nutritional status are at the borders of adequacy, periods of illness precipitate overt malnutrition and the patient enters a cycle of poor nutritional intake and repeated episodes of illness.

There is clearly some overlap between these classifications and it is also possible that some patients may be affected by more than one type concurrently. This classification may be useful in trying to decide upon the appropriate intervention for an individual. Thus a specific deficiency might be dealt with by inclusion of particular foods in the diet or even by the use of nutrient supplements. Sudden malnutrition might require intensive intervention until the medical or social problem has been resolved, whilst the longstanding malnutrition might be best helped by arranging long-term nutritional support such as the provision of community meals or even residential care.

The impact of nutritional support

There is a considerable body of evidence that nutritional supplementation has substantial beneficial effects upon outcome measures in both chronically, and acutely ill elderly people (see Chapter 8). Undernutrition is prevalent amongst elderly people in the community, in residential homes and those admitted to hospital, even for acute conditions. Undernutrition probably plays a role in precipitating both chronic and acute conditions as well as clearly exacerbating illness and slowing recovery. This means that any measures that improve the nutritional status of elderly people can be expected to yield substantial benefits in reducing mortality, reducing morbidity and increasing the quality of life of many elderly people.

In contrast to the quite extensive and growing literature dealing with the impact of nutritional support for elderly people in hospital, information about the impact of community meals, other home-based assistance and improved catering and feeding care in residential homes is lacking. It is therefore mainly assumption, largely based upon indirect evidence and extrapolation, that measures designed to improve the nutritional status of non-hospitalised elderly people will yield substantial health benefits for them and cost benefits for society as a whole. It is an assumption that we believe to be justified.

Measures to improve nutritional status

Webb (1995) has previously suggested some measures that might lead to a general improvement in the nutritional wellbeing of hospital patients. Table 7.1 shows an adaptation of this list to apply more specifically to elderly hospital patients. These measures or objectives could be applied to residential homes for the elderly almost without modification.

- Better nutrition knowledge and heightened nutrition awareness amongst residential home staff. A recognition that good nutrition is an important factor in determining the health and wellbeing of residents. An understanding of how the nutritional needs and priorities of some elderly residents might differ from those of younger adults.

Table 7.1 Measures that could improve the nutritional status of elderly hospitalised patients (modified after Webb, 1995)

1   Measures designed to heighten the awareness of medical and nursing staff to the importance of good nutrition to the health and wellbeing of elderly patients.
2   Improved training to help staff to recognise the signs of malnutrition and to better understand the nutrient needs of elderly hospital patients.
3   Provision of adequate amounts of appetising, acceptable and nutritious food that reaches patients in good condition. Table 5.8 in Chapter 5 highlights some of the service provision issues that may prevent this aim being fulfilled, e.g. lack of staff for feeding assistance and prolonged warm-holding of food leading to deterioration of both nutritional quality and palatability.
4   Assessment of patients on admission, to identify those already undernourished, and the institution of corrective measures where appropriate.
5   Routine monitoring of intakes (e.g. by noting plate waste) and anthropometric indicators of nutritional status (e.g. body weight). Use of more sophisticated indices of nutritional status, where appropriate.
6   Early introduction of intervention measures for those identified as malnourished. This may mean the involvement of dietitians or specialist nutrition nurses. The impact of nutritional interventions and supplementation in elderly hospital patients is dealt with in Chapter 8.

- Provision of residents with adequate amounts of nutritious and appetising food and ensuring that they are given sufficient time to eat and, where appropriate, all necessary assistance with eating. Maximising the choice of food offered to residents and maximising their involvement in menu design.
- Increased vigilance of staff, and formal procedures for detecting signs of malnutrition amongst residents. Nutritional assessment of all new residents. Regular weighing or other simple anthropometric measurement. Monitoring levels of plate waste and trying to ascertain reasons for high wastage.
- Access to, and readiness to use, a specialist nutrition/dietetic adviser when eating difficulties and nutritional problems arise.

Many of these measures or objectives could also be modified and/or generalised to make them relevant to the elderly population living in their own homes.

- All of those having medical or welfare contact with elderly people might benefit from increased education about nutrition and its importance to older people (e.g. general practitioners, health visitors, district nurses). Elderly people themselves, and friends and relatives concerned about their welfare, would benefit from increased awareness and improved understanding of the principles of good nutritional practice for the elderly.

- Increased vigilance on the part of medical and care workers for signs of deteriorating nutritional status or food intake. Some specific nutrition screening element could usefully be included in the annual screening of the over-75s discussed in Chapter 6. This would be made much more likely by the widespread acceptance of a very simple nutritional screening tool (see Chapter 6 for examples).
- Provision of adequate amounts of food and nutrients is clearly still a major priority in the community but measures to achieve this are much more complex and multi-faceted in free-living than in 'captive' populations. Identifying those who would benefit from and accept community meals has been dealt with in Chapter 6. It is also important that these community meals are of good nutritional quality, are palatable and reach the clients in good condition. Quality of community meals is dealt with later in this chapter. For many elderly people a variety of indirect measures may have significant nutritional impact, such as:

  - ensuring that they are aware of and claim all of their financial entitlements

  - providing assistance or transport for shopping

  - providing assistance with domestic chores

  - providing modified tools or utensils for preparing food or eating

  - access to a lunch club or community centre where food can be purchased and enjoyed in a social atmosphere.

- Ready access to community-based, nutrition/dietetics specialists and a willingness of other medical and care workers to use them.

One recurring theme that runs through these three sets of measures is the need for improved nutritional training and awareness of carers. This applies whether they are based in hospitals, residential homes or in the community.

Community meals

INTRODUCTION

The term community meals includes meals served at luncheon clubs and day centres for the elderly as well as meals delivered to people in their own homes – 'meals on wheels'. These community meals are not just valuable for nutritional support but they may also be an important source of social contact for elderly people who live alone.

According to CWT (1995), almost 33 million meals were served to elderly people in their own homes in the UK in 1992. Those elderly people receiving delivered meals tend to be the most vulnerable of those still able to live independently, principally those who are judged unable to provide a daily, hot main meal for themselves. This may be because of physical or mental incapacity or because of lack of access to adequate food preparation facilities. Provision of this service may be an important way of extending the period that an elderly person can remain living independently in their own home. However, it is important that 'meals on wheels' is not regarded as the automatic and only solution to any perceived nutritional problem. There may be other, cheaper alternatives that would serve the nutritional needs of the client just as well and might better serve their other needs, for example:

- arranging transport to a local lunch club
- arranging for home deliveries by local retailers
- arranging transport for shopping trips.

Other examples of these so-called 'enabling services' were given in Chapter 6.

Luncheon clubs and day centres can attract a wide range of elderly people – from the active, independent elderly through to those only able to attend if transport is provided. They are organised by a variety of charitable and statutory organisations and so it is extremely difficult to estimate either the number of lunch clubs or the number of meals that they provide; one UK charity (the Women's Royal Voluntary Service) operates around 1000 lunch clubs. Some community meals may also be provided in sheltered accommodation for the elderly; sheltered accommodation allows elderly people to live independently in their own self-contained apartment but with a warden on call when needed. Some of these complexes have communal dining areas and/or food preparation facilities (CWT, 1995).

Nutritional standards for community meals

An expert working party in the UK (CWT, 1995) has recently suggested some nutritional standards for community meals. It suggests that delivered 'meal packages' should consist of not only the main meal and dessert for immediate consumption but also a snack to be eaten later in the day. These standards indicate that the daily meal package should contain, on average, at least 33% of the RNI for elderly people for most essential nutrients but should supply higher proportions of the dietary standards for certain key nutrients, namely:

- 40% of the energy EAR
- 40% of the RNI for folate, calcium and iron
- 50% of the RNI for vitamin C.

The working party further recommends that the meal package should:

- contain 6 g of dietary fibre (non-starch polysaccharide) – a third of the DRV
- have 35% of the food energy as fat
- have 11% of the food energy as extrinsic non milk sugars
- have 39% of the food energy as starches and intrinsic sugars.

Table 7.2 gives an example of a meal package that could be delivered and that meets the CWT guidelines. It is not an excessively bulky meal and would hopefully be acceptable to most people receiving community meals. In the CWT (1995) report, there are more examples of suitable menus and their nutritional analyses. There are also examples of community meals suitable for

Table 7.2 An example of a meal package for home delivery to an elderly person that would meet the nutritional guidelines of CWT (1995). Data source: CWT (1995)

Quantity	Food
100 ml	Fruit juice
90 g	Roast pork
20 g	Apple sauce
60 g	Cabbage
45 g	Sweetcorn
90 g	Roast potatoes
90 g	Rhubarb crumble
90 g	Custard
Later snack	
50 g	Jam sponge

older people from the main ethnic minority communities in the UK. Some system for recording the views of clients and delivery staff about the quality and acceptability of the meals should be in place and used as feedback to adjust the meal provision according to the wishes of the clients.

Catering in residential and nursing homes

Overview

A large minority of elderly people live in some form of residential accommodation for the elderly (more than a quarter of the over 85s). These are people who, by definition, are no longer able to cope independently and thus tend to be the most vulnerable amongst the elderly population. Many have severe mobility difficulties or are suffering from dementia or some other mental deterioration, or are simply frail. More than two-thirds of residential places are in the private sector where profitability is naturally an important consideration of the management. Even though many profitable homes are well-managed and provide a very high standard of care for their residents, this situation clearly requires monitoring and vigilance on the part of the licensing authorities.

An expert working group (CWT, 1995) has recently published guideline standards for meals in residential and nursing homes and these are summarised later in the chapter. This group recommended that there should be regular monitoring of the standards of meals in residential and nursing homes. Failure to meet nutritional standards, should ultimately be grounds for rescinding of registration if advice on ways of improving standards proves ineffective. This group considered that at 1994 prices, at least £15 ($22.50) per resident per week needed to be spent on food ingredients to ensure an adequate and palatable diet; many homes at that time spent considerably less than this.

Assessment and monitoring

Admission to a residential or nursing home is often an unplanned event that can be extremely traumatic for the older person and leave them shocked and confused for some time after admission. Many people enter residential accommodation after discharge from hospital for an acute condition or a sudden deterioration of a chronic condition. During this early period, many new residents experience loss of appetite, apathy and a general feeling of despair. As part of the admissions procedure, there should be a thorough assessment of the new resident's nutritional status and dietary needs. The new resident should be weighed and any recent weight changes identified. Their food likes and dislikes and their particular dietary requirements should be determined and integrated into the care plan.

- Do they need a special therapeutic diet?
- Do they have any special cultural or religious dietary constraints?
- Do they have any intolerances or allergies?

With new residents, initially food and fluid intake should be monitored and the amount of plate waste recorded.,

Established residents should be weighed regularly (say monthly) and any unintentional weight loss noted, investigated and, where appropriate, treated.

Nutritional guidelines for residential and nursing homes for elderly people

CWT (1995) set the following nutritional guidelines for the average daily food provided for elderly people in residential and nursing homes. These guidelines are based upon the Dietary Reference Values published in COMA (1991) and these were discussed, at length, in Chapter 5.

- The food should provide at least the EAR for energy appropriate to the person's age and sex.
- The food should provide amounts of the major essential nutrients (i.e. for protein, thiamin (B_1), riboflavin (B_2), niacin (B_3), folate, vitamin C, vitamin A, calcium, iron, sodium and potassium) that are equal to, or exceed the RNI.
- The food should provide an average 18 g/day of dietary fibre (non-starch polysaccharide).

- 35% of the food energy should come from fat, 39% from starch and intrinsic sugars, and 11% from non-milk extrinsic sugars.
- Residents who do not get regular access to sunlight may need vitamin D supplements.

The assumption would be that any menu plan meeting these standards would almost inevitably contain adequate amounts of all of the other essential nutrients that are not specifically listed.

Menu planning

CWT (1995) give an example of a typical week's menus for older people living in residential accommodation that would meet the nutritional guidelines that they set and which were listed in the previous section. An example of a single day's menu from this report is shown in Table 7.3.

NAGE (1992) set some general dietary targets in the form of daily food portions and these are shown in Table 7.4.

It is important that a menu plan is prepared by the cook. Not only must the food offered be adequate and meet the nutritional criteria listed but it must also be eaten by the clients. It must, therefore, also look and taste pleasant; there should be interesting combinations and the residents should be offered as much choice as possible. Residents should have an input into the menu plan, they should be able to make sure that favourite dishes are included and make suggestions particularly for special occasions like Easter and Christmas.

One practical point to consider in any bulk catering situation is that the water soluble vitamins are relatively heat labile (B vitamins, folic acid and vitamin C). In order to maximise their retention in the food eaten then the following precautions need to be taken:

- good quality fresh or frozen vegetables should be used
- the vegetables should not be cut too finely and should not be overcooked
- vegetables should be served as soon after cooking as possible.

High quality frozen vegetables are likely to have higher nutrient content than poor quality fresh vegetables or those delivered only once or twice a week.

Timing of meals

The timing of meals is an important factor in determining the food and nutrient intakes of residents. As far as possible, the residents' preferences should be taken into account in meal timing, for example would they prefer their main meal in the evening or at lunchtime? It is common practice for residents to have a cooked breakfast, lunch as the main meal and then a relatively light evening meal; this is often convenient for catering staff and may well reproduce the traditional practices of many retired people. If this practice is adopted, spacing of the meals is an important consideration – the main meal

Table 7.3 An example of a day's menu for older people living in residential or nursing homes. This is part of a weekly menu plan that meets the nutritional standards of CWT (1995). Data source: The Caroline Walker Trust (1995)

Breakfast

Prunes (100 g)
Porridge made with milk from allowance (150 g) or high fibre cereal (45 g), with milk from allowance
Toast (white or wholemeal) (40 g) with butter/margarine from allowance and marmalade or jam (20 g)
Tea or coffee with milk

Mid morning

Tea/coffee with milk and digestive biscuit (15 g)

Lunch

Fruit juice (100 ml)
Chicken fricasee (120 g)
Carrots (60 g)
Broccoli (60 g)
Mashed potato (100 g)
Apple pie (90 g)
Custard (90 g)

Mid afternoon

Tea/coffee with milk
Fruit scone (60 g) with butter/margarine

Evening meal

Scrambled egg (100 g)
Toast (40 g) and butter/margarine
Chocolate eclair (45 g)
Banana (90 g)

Bedtime

Milky drink made with milk allowance

Daily allowances

600 ml (about a pint) of semi-skimmed milk
20 g butter or polyunsaturated margarine

should not be too close to the cooked breakfast and the final evening meal should not be too early. In the A–Z checklist for assessing residential homes (described in Chapter 6) one of the factors identified as increasing the risk of nutritional deficiency is serving the final evening meal before 5 p.m. Serving the evening meal too early leaves a very long gap between the final evening

Table 7.4 Dietary targets for menus in residential accommodation for the elderly. Data source: NAGE (1992)

Try to Include each day: Food	Quantity
Milk	0.5–1 pint each day (more if person is not eating)
Select 2 portions from: Meat Fish Cheese Eggs	cooked weight 50–75 g portion 100–125 g portion 50 g portion 1 egg
Bread, Rice, Pasta Breakfast cereals, Potatoes	Provide 1 or more helpings of these at each meal. Amounts will vary with appetite.
Vegetables (fresh, frozen or salad)	At least 2 portions daily
Fruit (fresh, dried, stewed, tinned, fruit juice)	1 portion daily
Fluids (tea, coffee, fruit juice, soup, water etc.)	At least 8 cups daily

meal and breakfast. Such bunching of meals may be very attractive from a staffing viewpoint because all of the meals can be prepared within a normal working day. However, this bunching will probably depress the total food intake of residents, especially of those whose appetite is not good.

Ensuring adequate fluid intakes was identified in Chapter 3 as an important consideration in the care of the elderly; ideally residents should consume eight cups of fluid per day. Mid-morning and mid-afternoon drinks should be part of normal routine and where possible a choice of drinks should be offered. A choice of drinks should be easily available to residents at all times. The more mobile residents could have access to tea and coffee making facilities and perhaps be encouraged to be involved in drink making and distribution for the other residents.

Serving of meals

Table 7.5 gives a summary of some of the things to be considered when organising and serving meals in residential and nursing homes. The general aim in arranging the dining area should be to produce an environment that as nearly as possible resembles that in an older person's own home. It should be a friendly, welcoming and culturally appropriate place, perhaps with flowers on the table. Condiments and sauces should be available and on the table. Some residents may need to be supplied with aids such as non-slip mats or wide-handled spoons to enable them to eat their meal independently. Where assistance is required it should be given discretely, if at all possible; it should be offered cheerfully and unhurriedly and the assistant should do all they can to avoid damaging the dignity and self-esteem of the resident.

Some other points

Anything that makes the atmosphere of the residential home more like a normal home should help to maintain the morale and self-esteem of residents, for example:

* some homes have a snack bar or small shop where snacks, toiletries and alcoholic or soft drinks can be purchased by residents
* some homes arrange regular trips for residents to cafes, restaurants or for fish and chips

Table 7.5 Factors to consider in the service of meals in residential and nursing homes

Physical environment

Seating arrangement
Chairs of appropriate height and type
Appropriate cutlery
Noise level
Distractions
Avoid offensive odours

Social environment

Sufficient time allocated for eating
Compatibility of dining companions
Personal preferences, e.g. resident who wishes to eat alone
Pleasant and non-patronising serving staff
Appropriate and discrete assistance

Meal

Portion size
Appearance
Taste, smell, colour and texture
Individual likes and dislikes
Familiarity and cultural acceptability
Temperature
Second helping available
Sufficient fluid (tea, coffee, fruit juice, water etc.)

- residents can be encouraged to invite guests in for small meals or drinks and biscuits
- special events, such as birthdays, can be marked by celebration-type food and drink.

It is important for staff to remember that residential and nursing homes are the homes of the residents and not a place of confinement and management. The elderly residents should be afforded as much freedom of movement and even the freedom to partly cater for themselves as is consistent with the proper management of the home and the safety of its residents.

The benefits of physical activity to older people have been discussed at some length in Chapters 3 and 4. Even very elderly people have been shown to gain substantial benefits from training programmes (Fiatarone et al., 1994). Elderly people should be encouraged to maintain physical activity by doing everyday things like walking. For those residents who wish it, the availability of some more formal programme of appropriate exercises would be a useful for maintaining, or even improving, physical wellbeing, improving their self-esteem and as a social activity.

A note about hospital catering

The issue of catering in hospitals has not been specifically addressed in this chapter; this is an issue of importance to hospital residents of all ages and is not an issue particular to elderly people. Much of what has been said about nutrition and eating in residential homes would be equally applicable to hospitals. In general, the nutritional standards for nursing and residential homes for the elderly, published in CWT (1995), could be applied to hospital menus for the elderly. However, it should be borne in mind that there is a high probability that the food intake of elderly hospital patients will be depressed by a variety of factors such as those listed in Table 5.6. Illness and injury may also increase the need for energy and/or nutrients because of nutrient losses or because of increased nutrient turnover (see Table 5.6). The Dietary Reference Values (COMA, 1991), upon which the nutritional standards of CWT (1995) are based, are intended for use with healthy people and take no account of any increased requirement for energy and nutrients associated with disease or injury.

Ensuring the microbiological safety of food for the elderly (adapted from Webb, 1995)

There is a particular need to ensure the microbiological safety of food produced by those catering for the elderly for the reasons listed below.

- There is a decline in immunocompetence and increased susceptibility to infection in the elderly. Reduced gastric acid secretion may also make elderly people more prone to foodborne infections.

- There is increased severity of illness and slower recovery in the elderly because of these age-related changes in the immune system.
- Elderly people, and especially the frail elderly, have reduced ability to tolerate bouts of acute illness. Bouts of illness will worsen nutritional status.
- All mass catering situations have the potential to cause very large numbers of individual cases of food poisoning.

Frail, elderly people may suffer serious illness or even death from doses of organisms that would not affect or produce only mild illness in young, healthy people. Over the period 1979–1989, notification rates for food poisoning more than tripled amongst the elderly population of England and Wales (DH, 1992a). These changes in the apparent incidence of food poisoning essentially parallel the increases seen in younger age groups over this period. Food poisoning is rarely recorded as a cause of death, even amongst the elderly. In 1992, only 240 deaths in England and Wales were attributed to all intestinal infectious diseases (ICD codes 001–009) but 82% of these deaths occurred in people over 65 years of age.

Some organisms that cause foodborne infections have a very low infective dose; only a few organisms need be ingested to produce illness (e.g. the organisms responsible for typhoid, paratyphoid, Shigella dysentery and cholera). In these cases, contamination of food with the organism or even the presence of a few organisms in drinking water is enough to produce illness. However, with most of the common food poisoning organisms, large numbers of organisms need to be present in the food to produce illness. These common food poisoning organisms are said to have a high infective dose. With these organisms, not only must the food be contaminated but the bacteria need to multiply in the food before they represent a real hazard to the healthy consumer. Hundreds of thousands or even millions of bacteria may be needed to produce illness in healthy young adults. The infective dose may be at least an order of magnitude less in frail and very elderly people.

In order to grow within food, bacteria need nutrients, moisture, a favourable chemical environment, a suitable temperature and time to grow. These requirements make some foods unlikely causes of food poisoning, for example:

- dry foods like bread and biscuits lack the necessary moisture for bacterial growth and in very salty or sugary foods (e.g. jam), the water is unavailable to bacteria (moulds will still grow on these foods)
- the high acidity of some foods, like pickles, prevents bacterial growth
- fruits and vegetables lack the nutrients necessary for bacterial growth
- bacteria will not grow in oils and fats, like butter and margarine.

These foods can however act as sources of contamination for other foods. Commercially canned, sterilised or pasteurised foods are also highly unlikely to cause food poisoning if eaten immediately after opening because the commercial heat treatment kills all potential pathogens.

Meat, poultry, eggs, fish and shellfish are rich in the nutrients that bacteria need for growth, they have high water contents and have a pH conducive to rapid bacterial growth. Meat, poultry and eggs are the foods most commonly associated with food poisoning in the UK. These foods need to be handled and prepared with particular care. In an analysis of a large number of UK food poisoning outbreaks, Roberts (1982) identified a number of factors that were commonly associated with these outbreaks, including:

- preparation of food in advance of needs
- storage at room temperature
- inadequate heating or cooling
- undercooking
- inadequate thawing
- cross-contamination between foods
- improper warm-holding of food
- an infected food handler
- use of leftovers.

The three general aims below are crucial to ensuring the microbiological safety of food prepared for the elderly.

MINIMISE THE RISKS OF BACTERIAL CONTAMINATION

For example:

- buy food that is fresh and from suppliers who store and prepare it hygienically
- keep food covered and protected from insect contamination
- wash hands thoroughly before preparing food and after using the toilet or blowing one's nose
- cover any infected lesions on hands
- ensure that all utensils and surfaces that come into contact with food are clean
- ensure that any cloth used to clean utensils and surfaces or to dry dishes is clean and changed regularly
- avoid any contact between raw food (especially meat) and cooked food
- wash utensils, hands and surfaces in contact with raw food before they are used with cooked food.

MAXIMISE THE KILLING OF BACTERIA DURING FOOD PREPARATION

For example:

- cook meat, poultry and eggs thoroughly so that all parts of the food reach a minimum of 75°C
- defrost frozen meat and poultry thoroughly before cooking
- meat eaten 'rare' will not have undergone sufficient heat treatment to kill all bacteria and represents a hazard if contaminated prior to cooking, poultry should always be well-cooked
- raw eggs (e.g. in home-made mayonnaise) and undercooked eggs represent a potential hazard to the elderly
- when food is re-heated it should be thoroughly re-heated so that all parts of it reach 75°C.

MINIMISE THE TIME THAT FOOD IS STORED UNDER CONDITIONS THAT PERMIT BACTERIAL GROWTH

For example:

- food should be prepared as close to the time of consumption as is practical (prolonged holding of food also leads to loss of nutrients)
- when food is prepared well in advance of preparation it should be protected from contamination and not stored at room temperature
- discard foods that are past their 'use by' date or show evidence of spoilage (e.g. 'off' flavours and smells or discolouration)
- food that is kept hot should be kept at 65°C or above
- food that is kept cool should be kept below 5°C
- when food is cooked for storage it should be cooled quickly
- leftovers or other prepared foods that are stored in a refrigerator should be covered and used promptly.

Nutrition as therapy in sick elderly people

Introduction and scope of the chapter

The first part of this chapter deals with the management of individuals with a range of eating difficulties and the various strategies and devices that are available to maintain the flow of energy and essential nutrients to such patients. The second part of the chapter deals with the role of diet in the management of five specific conditions that are very common in the elderly. In four of these conditions, diet and nutritional factors are thought to be important in the aetiology of the condition as well as in its management. These five conditions are so prevalent amongst the elderly that anyone involved in caring for the elderly will have clients affected by them.

The aim of this chapter is to give non-specialists enough awareness and understanding of the dietary therapies to enable them to give practical support and encouragement to their clients and thus to help them comply with any prescribed diet. It may also help them to recognise when referral for specialist dietetic help or advice might be appropriate. The discussion is restricted to concepts and principles, such as:

- the rationale and justification for dietary intervention

- the dietary goals and strategies for achieving them
- evidence of the effectiveness of dietary management.

Detailed dietetic instructions and diet plans are beyond the scope of this book and are the province of the specialist dietitian and specialist manuals of dietetic practice (e.g. Thomas, 1994).

One general principle that applies to any diet is that there must always be a balance between what may be theoretically desirable and what is acceptable and achievable. With encouragement, many elderly people will modify their food and fluid intake, but advice to make unrealistically extreme changes may lessen the chances of any beneficial changes being made. It is a relatively straightforward matter to devise diets or plan menus that meet any particular set of compositional criteria. It is a much more difficult task to produce menus that are also acceptable to the recipients. It seems reasonable to expect that diets in sympathy with the preferences and usual selection practices of the clients will have the best chance of achieving good compliance.

Dietary management of patients with eating difficulties

Low body weight is a predictor of subsequent mortality in elderly people (Exton-Smith, 1988). Low food intake not only leads to weight loss, but also increases the probability that the intake of other nutrients will be inadequate; the severe consequences of malnutrition during illness and injury and in otherwise healthy people have been dealt with earlier. This section deals with a number of problems that, if untreated, are likely to result in weight loss and nutrient deficiency in elderly people. Undernutrition and its consequences can be avoided in many elderly people by the appropriate use of nutritional supplements and artificial feeding methods. Greater awareness of the range and effectiveness of these nutritional support measures could play a part in reducing the high prevalence of malnutrition amongst sick elderly people.

The problems

A number of problems may cause older people to have difficulty consuming adequate amounts of food energy and/or nutrients.

SMALL APPETITE

Many older people have a reduced appetite. In some cases, there may be a discernible explanation, such as a medical condition, a mental problem, or a medical treatment that causes anorexia. In many other cases there is no such obvious cause. In Chapter 3, clear evidence was presented that ageing results in a reduced acuity of the thirst response to dehydration which compounds with other problems (e.g. fetching drinks) to substantially increase the risk of dehydration. One might suggest, by analogy, that there may be a similar decline in the sensitivity of the hunger mechanism to body energy stores, thus making the elderly more prone to undernutrition in the same way as they are more prone to dehydration. In such circumstances, it is important to encourage small, regular meals and snacks. Evidence that has been reviewed in Chapter 3 suggests that regular offering of drinks can greatly reduce the risks of dehydration in the elderly. Reduced intake of food energy may make it difficult for older people to meet their requirements for other nutrients. It is therefore important that the diet of people consuming small total amounts of food is nutrient dense (that it has high levels of nutrients per unit of energy).

DRY MOUTH

This is often a side effect of medication or illness. Fizzy drinks before a meal can refresh the mouth; chewing ice cubes may be helpful in stimulating saliva production. Artificial saliva can be prescribed which will enable the person to lubricate their food.

SORE MOUTH

A sore mouth can be caused by ill-fitting dentures, an infection, such as thrush, or it may be related to some other medical condition. Treatment for the cause of the sore mouth is clearly a priority, but some modification in the type of food offered may also be needed in the short-term, or in the longer term if the underlying cause proves refractory to treatment. Acidic fruits, hot foods and spicy foods may well tend to aggravate the condition.

NAUSEA

Nausea is a common symptom of many illnesses and is a side effect of many drugs and of radiotherapy. Constipation may also cause nausea. Strong cooking odours or other smells may exacerbate the problem.

DENTAL HEALTH

The majority of elderly people in the UK are still edentulous even though this situation is improving as more people are retaining at least some of their natural teeth well into old age. The state of dentition will have an impact upon the ability to chew, to swallow and may have a large restricting effect upon the range of foods eaten. Given the historical assumption that most elderly people have no natural teeth, regular dental checking and maintenance may be overlooked in the elderly.

SWALLOWING DIFFICULTIES – DYSPHAGIA

The normal swallow is a complex chain of neurological events. It may be divided into three phases:

The oral phase. The teeth and lips close and the food is formed into a bolus and moved by the tongue to the back of the mouth. This phase is a voluntary process, whereas the subsequent stages are reflex events.

The pharyngeal phase. The presence of food in the pharynx stimulates pressure receptors there which, in turn, leads to activation of a swallowing centre in the medulla of the brain. This swallowing centre sends out effector signals that bring about the complex sequence of muscle contractions and relaxations that make up the rest of the swallowing process. The soft palate rises and closes the nasopharynx so that the food is not regurgitated into the nasal cavities. The larynx (vocal cords) rises and the glottis closes to prevent the food entering the airway. A flap of tissue, the epiglottis, tilts downwards to cover the closed glottis.

The oesophageal phase. The upper oesophageal sphincter relaxes which enables the bolus of food to pass through the oesophagus and into the stomach.

Each stage triggers the next phase. A breakdown anywhere in the chain can interfere with food intake and affect nutritional status. Different textures of foods pass through the system at different rates; liquids are passed through the system more quickly than solids and so, for example, many dysphagic patients experience particular difficulty with drinking liquids because they reach the back of the mouth before the entrance to the trachea is blocked.

An abnormality in swallowing can lead to malnutrition and/or dehydration. There is a wide range of swallowing problems which can cause a variety of eating difficulties, such as:

- choking, airway obstruction and aspiration of food or drink into the lungs
- nasal regurgitation of food or drink
- dribbling of liquids resulting from an inadequate lip seal
- reduced ability to manipulate food in the mouth because of loss of sensation and poor control of the tongue.

Dysphagia is not a normal part of ageing, it is a secondary consequence of a disease process (e.g. stroke). An older person may, however, have a reduced ability to adapt and compensate for an inadequate swallow; reduced saliva production and chewing difficulties in the elderly may also increase swallowing difficulties. In the UK, patients with swallowing difficulties are usually referred to a speech and language therapist for diagnosis and management of their particular swallowing difficulties.

Some solutions

SUPPLEMENTS

A nutritional supplement is any item that is given in addition to the ordinary diet in order to increase the energy and/or nutrient intake of an inadequately nourished person. There are several types of supplements that can be used.

- **A snack between meals,** such as a milky drink between breakfast and lunch.
- **Enrichment** of an ordinary food with another energy and/or nutrient-dense food that does not increase the volume of the meal (e.g. milk powder added to ordinary milk or butter/margarine added to potatoes).

- **A dietary supplement,** e.g. the well known commercial products like *Complan* (Nestlé) and *Build Up* (Crookes Healthcare). They are concentrated energy and/or nutrient sources that are usually consumed in liquid form and are readily digested and absorbed. Crowther (1989) has reviewed the use of these supplements in the elderly and classifies them into four categories:

  - **protein and energy/meal supplements** – these are based on skimmed milk powder or milk protein (casein), they are fortified with vitamins and minerals and may have added fibre. Some are in the form of powders that are designed to be mixed with water to form a supplementary drink and some come in the form of puddings. They have wide suitability, e.g. for most patients at risk of, or suffering from undernutrition for many of the reasons listed above.
  - **protein supplements** – based upon milk or soya protein. They come in the form of soup or dessert mixes or as powders designed to be added to other foods particularly suitable for patients with low blood protein concentrations.
  - **carbohydrate supplements** – based upon glucose polymers but they are much less sweet than sugar. These are used for patients who require additional energy without added bulk. They are often in powder form and can be incorporated into other foods and drinks without much effect on the taste.
  - **fat supplements** – fat emulsions that may be combined with glucose polymers and used to boost the energy content of low protein diets (e.g. in renal failure). Some are made from a highly refined and easily absorbed type of fat (medium chain triglycerides) and these are designed for patients with malabsorption.

The use of supplements needs to be monitored and subjected to regular review, particularly the impact of the supplement on other food and fluid consumption. Sometimes the addition of energy or nutrient-rich foods to the diet is more appropriate and acceptable to patients than the use of commercial supplements that are sometimes rather unpalatable. Dehydration is a potential danger if the total fluid is not monitored.

- **Micronutrient supplements** – concentrated sources of individual vitamins or minerals or multinutrient supplements. In some cases micronutrient supplements may be the most practical way of ensuring adequacy of these nutrients in some elderly patients. In patients whose total food intake is very low, because of low energy expenditure and poor appetite, major changes in the diet designed to boost the nutrient density may simply reduce food intake still further and precipitate energy deficit. In elderly housebound people, supplements are the only practical way of achieving a regular vitamin D intake of 10 µg/day (the UK RNI for this group).

CHANGES IN THE TEXTURE OF FOOD

Texture of food is very important to its palatability and generally meals should consist of a variety of different textures. Textures of food have been classified by dietitians and speech therapists depending on the ease of consumption (Table 8.1). In some medical conditions, the texture of food needs to be modified, for example:

- problems in the mouth such as ill fitting dentures or cancer of the mouth
- problems with the swallow reflex
- physical obstruction (e.g. oesophageal stricture or obstruction)
- some psychiatric disorders
- neurological changes (e.g. after a stroke).

Table 8.1 A classification of food textures with food examples

Texture classification	Example of food
Hard	Apple
Chewy	Cooked meat
Soft	Cake, bread/butter (no crust)
Liquid hard lump	Muesli
Liquid soft lump	Cornflakes & milk
Thickened soft lump	Plain yoghurt & banana
Thickened hard lump	Stew with chewy meat
Liquid	Milk, water & orange juice
Slide down easy	Butter, peanut butter, mousse

The oral feeding of dysphagic patients will be used to illustrate this use of changes in diet texture.

The correct feeding position is very important for dysphagic patients. The head should be in mid-line with the spine and the neck must not be extended or over-flexed. Extra time must also be allowed for feeding dysphagic patients, as rushing can be an additional source of tension.

The degree of dysphagia will determine the degree to which the texture of the diet needs to be manipulated. The following are examples of the types of diet that might be offered to patients with progressively worse levels of dysphagia:

- a soft diet using minced meat, flaked fish, soft vegetables, mashed potatoes, soft fruit (without skin), milk puddings, bread and butter (no crust)
- a soft smooth diet where the food is soft and mashed, for example pureed meat, mashed soft vegetables, soft mashed potatoes, mashed soft fruit and milk pudding

- a pureed diet where food is pureed using a blender and additional water added, such as pureed meat, pureed potato, pureed vegetables, smooth yoghurt, mousse and ground rice pudding.

As the degree of restriction increases so the likelihood of an inadequate intake increases. When food is pureed with extra fluid, it becomes more dilute and often acquires a watery taste and unacceptable appearance. If a whole meal is liquidised, the appearance of the resulting mixture is often revolting and bears little resemblance in appearance or taste to the original. This is not recommended. Patients who require pureed food are likely to have an inadequate energy intake and therefore they often require supplementation to prevent malnutrition.

As has already been stated, liquids can present particular problems to some dysphagic patients because they may reach the back of the mouth too quickly, before the airway has been blocked. A number of thickening agents have been produced commercially; these are powders which can be stirred into a liquid to make it thicker and easier to swallow.

ARTIFICIAL FEEDING

For some patients, it may not be possible to maintain an adequate supply of energy and nutrients via the normal oral route. In such cases some form of artificial feeding will be required, either as a supplement to the oral intake or as a total replacement for it. This would include patients with severe dysphagia where severe risk of aspiration precludes use of the normal oral route. Artificial feeding may be subdivided into enteral and parenteral feeding.

Enteral feeding. Nutrients are passed directly into the stomach by use of a tube that is introduced through the nose and into the stomach: a nasogastric tube. Sometimes this tube may empty directly into the intestine and tubes introduced directly into the gut by surgical means are also used. KFC (1992) estimated that around 2% of hospitalised patients in Britain receives some form of artificial feeding and that in three-quarters of cases an enteral tube is the method used. Strict hygiene practices must be maintained whenever tube feeding is used. Some common problems associated with nasogastric feeding:

- the tube may be pulled out by the patient
- discomfort caused by the tube irritating the nose or oesophagus
- blockage of the tube (the tube needs to be flushed at regular intervals and a dilute solution of sodium bicarbonate will often dissolve a blockage)
- reflux of gastric contents and possible aspiration because the gastro-oesophageal sphincter is held open (the risk can be reduced if the patient is sat up with their head elevated and the rate of feeding is not too fast)
- aspiration of saliva
- diarrhoea.

For long term artificial feeding of elderly people in the community, then gastrostomy feeding is becoming more widely used; that is a tube that has been inserted directly into the stomach by surgical means. It has a number of advantages over nasogastric feeding:

- it is more discrete
- there is no irritation of the nose or oesophagus
- it does not interfere with rehabilitation of normal swallowing or speech
- it can be left in place for several months.

Parenteral feeding. The patient may be supplied with nutrients intravenous-ly, either as a supplement to the oral route or as the sole means of nutrition (total parenteral nutrition or TPN). In TPN, the nutrients must be infused via an indwelling catheter into a large vein. In some cases of extreme damage to the gut, patients may be fed for years by TPN. A major factor that has enabled patients to be maintained indefinitely with TPN was the development of a means of safely infusing a source of fat intravenously.

Ideally these artificial feeding methods should be managed by a specialist nutrition team. Discussion of the practical details is beyond the scope of this book but interested readers may find further information in Grant and Todd (1987) or Taylor and Goodinson-McClaren (1992). TPN in particular, requires specialist management and is usually only used where the enteral route is ruled out, for example in patients who have had a large part of the intestine removed or have severe inflammatory disease of the intestine. Infection of the intravenous lines can be a major problem in TPN but with skilled specialist management it can be largely eliminated (KFC, 1992).

The effectiveness of nutritional support

COSTS

Supplementary feeding by the oral route is by far the cheapest way of increas-ing the flow of nutrients to patients. Whatever mode of supplementation is chosen the cost is likely to be only a few pounds per week on top of the £20 per week allowed for feeding a National Health Service patient in the UK. Use of enteral feeding will raise the cost of feeding the patient by several-fold and the costs of total parenteral feeding will be several hundred pounds per week, considerably more than an order of magnitude greater than the costs of oral feeding. For many patients who are undernourished or at risk of becoming undernourished, using supplements or artificial feeding to maintain or improve nutritional status is cost effective not only because of the benefits it yields for the patient, but also because it reduces the costs of coping with con-sequences of inadequate nutrition such as:

- higher infection rates
- slower healing
- slower re-mobilisation and increased duration of dependency
- longer hospital stay.

Selecting the lowest and, therefore, the cheapest level of intervention that will meet the needs of the patient will obviously optimise the costs to benefit ratio. Dietary intervention should be used to improve and/or extend life but such intervention cannot be justified if it merely prolongs the process of dying, e.g. TPN for patients with end-stage terminal disease. Figure 8.1 shows an outline scheme that could be used by an experienced dietitian or other nutrition specialist to decide upon the level of support that is appropriate for any given patient.

KFC (1992) has estimated that the potential financial savings that might accrue in the UK from a nationwide introduction of nutritional support for undernourished patients at over £250 ($375) million at 1992 prices.

Question 1	**Is the patient malnourished?**
Response	*Action*
No	No immediate action but continue to monitor and review.
Yes	Proceed to question 2
Question 2	**Can the patient tolerate ordinary foods in sufficient quantities to meet their needs?**
Response	*Action*
No	Proceed to question 3.
Yes	Check that the current level of service is adequate and make adjustments as deemed necessary, e.g. check that the patient is being offered sufficient food, that the food is appropriate in composition and texture and that the patient is receiving adequate time and assistance with feeding. Review the initial decision if the patient fails to make progress.
Question 3	**Would oral supplements help this patient?**
Response	*Action*
No	Proceed to question 4.
Yes	Arrange for appropriate supplements to be provided. Choose the lowest level of intervention that is likely to be effective and make sure that any supplementary product is appropriate for the condition. Monitor progress and review the initial decision if necessary.
Question 4	**Is the gut functioning sufficiently for enteral nutrition?**
Response	*Action*
No	Consider use of total parenteral nutrition (TPN). TPN is indicated if the problem is likely to be short term or if long term therapy is likely to offer the patient an improved quality of life and/or extension of life of reasonable quality. TPN is not indicated if it merely prolongs a very uncomfortable existence in patients with end stage terminal disease.
Yes	If intervention is appropriate (as above for TPN) initiate the appropriate form of enteral feeding, e.g. nasogastric tube, monitor progress and if necessary review the decision.

Figure 8.1 A scheme for deciding the appropriate level of nutritional support for a patient. Based on a scheme by Woods in RCN (1993)

BENEFITS

In many acute conditions, nutritional support can substantially reduce mortality. A number of controlled studies on the effects of supplementary feeding in hospital patients have been conducted and several of these have used elderly patients. Reduced complication rates, decreased length of hospital stay and reduced mortality rates are general findings from such studies (briefly reviewed by KFC, 1992).

One concern about the use of supplements is that they may depress the intake of other foods and thus act as substitutes rather than supplements, resulting in no net improvement in energy intake. In such a situation, unless supplements are nutrient-enriched they might actually depress nutrient intakes. Several studies have demonstrated that elderly patients who are given supplements do increase their overall energy intakes and/or show anthropometric indications of improved nutritional status (e.g. McEvoy and James, 1982; Elmstabl and Steen, 1987; Brown and Seabrook, 1992; Reilly et al., 1995). In a recent study of acutely ill and undernourished elderly patients, Reilly et al. (1995) have reported that three separate 100 ml sip feeds (1.5 kcal/ml) administered at the time of drug rounds had no effect upon voluntary energy intake and thus resulted in a 50% increase in total energy intake. Woo et al. (1994) gave supplements to a randomly selected sample of patients discharged from hospital after acute chest infections. These supplements were sufficient to cover only the first month after discharge but the supplemented patients still had anthropometric indications of better nutritional status than the control group at three months after discharge; they also had better status for some micronutrients. Elmstabl and Steel (1987) found that, prior to supplementation a sample of 28 women admitted to long stay geriatric care had very low energy intakes and evidence of inadequate intakes of specific micronutrients. The effects of three different supplements upon total food and nutrient intake and nutritional status were investigated. All three supplements resulted in a substantial increase in total energy intake (about 25%) and weight gain. The supplements had little effect upon normal food intake. There was some reduction in energy obtained from low nutrient density snacks. The supplement with the lowest volume resulted in the largest increase in total energy intake and the lowest suppression of appetite (i.e.the lowest reduction in normal food intake).

Larsson et al. (1990) carried out a randomised study of the effects of energy supplements using 500 patients admitted to a long stay geriatric ward of a Swedish hospital. The supplements reduced the deterioration in nutritional status following admission and reduced the mortality rate.

Two studies on the effects of supplementation in elderly patients with hip fractures suggest that oral or enteral (nasogastric tube) supplements improve both the nutritional status of the patients and measures of outcome. Supplementation was associated with reduced hospital stay, more rapid mobilisation, reduced rates of complications and lower mortality (Delmi et al., 1990; Bastow et al., 1983).

Dietary management of specific problems and diseases

The choice of conditions

Diet plays a role in the treatment of many diseases that affect both young and old. In this part of the chapter, we have selected a small number of conditions that are particularly prevalent amongst the elderly and thus some understanding is important for those charged with the care of the elderly. The conditions are:

- constipation
- diabetes mellitus
- obesity
- hyperlipidaemia
- dementia.

One of the authors (JC) surveyed 50 dietitians specialising in the care of the elderly about the most common reasons for referral and the problems most identified by the dietitians in their clients. Problems of anorexia, eating difficulties and weight loss were collectively the most prevalent and together they accounted for about a third of referrals; this has been dealt with in the first part of this chapter. Diabetes, obesity and constipation were the next most commonly mentioned in this survey and this is the justification for their inclusion in our list.

The hyperlipidaemias are included because of their prevalence amongst the elderly and because diet plays a major part in their treatment and in their aetiology. Around a quarter of elderly British women have plasma cholesterol concentrations that fall within the range normally classified as hypercholesteraemic. We have also included a short section dealing with the role of diet in the management of dementia patients. As the very elderly population of industrialised countries has grown, so the prevalence of dementia has increased and looks set to carry on increasing for the foreseeable future; dementia patients are frequently malnourished.

Constipation

INTRODUCTION

Constipation is defined as the passage of hard stools less frequently than normal for a particular individual. It is the commonest disorder of the gastrointestinal tract in older people and is especially prevalent in those with reduced mobility. According to Kassianos (1993) it accounts for 13 consultations per year for every 1000 patients on a general practitioners's list.

Constipation occurs more frequently in people with medical conditions that reduce mobility, reduce fluid intake or increase fluid loss. For example:

- in stroke and arthritis patients because of their reduced mobility
- in patients with fever because of increased fluid losses
- in patients with memory loss and terminal disease because of reduced fluid intake.

Constipation is a side-effect of several prescribed drugs including the narcotic analgesics (e.g. codeine and morphine).

More generally, ageing is associated with decreased physical activity, reduced fluid intake and increased fluid losses. More direct, age-related changes in the intestinal tract are also likely to increase the prevalence of constipation in the elderly (Chapter 3).

TREATMENT

Health professionals usually rely upon pharmacological means for treating constipation, e.g. laxatives and suppositories or the use of enemas. The alternative method of management is to try to reduce some of the underlying causes by increasing fluid intake, ensuring an adequate intake of dietary fibre and encouraging mobility.

In an unpublished 1992 survey conducted on 'care of the elderly' wards in Leeds hospitals, about 50% of admissions were receiving some form of regular treatment for constipation. Subsequent to this survey an education programme was introduced on some of the wards that was aimed at reducing the prevalence of constipation and a reduction in laxative use. The basic strategies of this programme were:

- to try to increase the fluid consumption of patients to at least eight cups a day
- to improve the toileting arrangements (e.g. more frequent offers by staff of toilet use)
- to try to increase the consumption of fruit and vegetables
- use of high fibre white or wholemeal bread.

These measures resulted in a marked reduction in the prevalence of constipation. The subsequent evaluation highlighted the importance of staff training to increase awareness of the problem and of some of the non-pharmacological solutions.

The general strategy for the dietary treatment and prevention of constipation is thus to:

- increase the fluid intake to at least eight full cups of liquid (non-alcoholic) a day
- increase the amount of dietary fibre from cereals, vegetable and fruit
- encourage increased physical activity.

DIETARY FIBRE OR NON-STARCH POLYSACCHARIDE (NSP)

Dietary fibre (NSP) consists of a range of different carbohydrate substances that act as structural components of plant cell walls (cellulose and hemicellulose) and viscous soluble substances found in cell sap of plants (pectin and gums); animal foods contain no dietary fibre. The term dietary fibre would also encompass lignin, a woody non-carbohydrate material and resistant starch (explanation below) but in this text the terms 'dietary fibre' and 'NSP' are used synonymously. All of the non-starch polysaccharides are resistant to digestion by human gut enzymes and therefore pass through the small intestine and into the large bowel undigested.

Dietary fibre is subdivided into two major fractions – the soluble substances (soluble fibre/NSP) that form gums and gels when mixed with water (the gums and pectins) and the water insoluble fraction (cellulose and hemicellulose). The insoluble forms of fibre predominate in the bran of wheat, rice and maize but rye, barley and particularly oats contain higher proportions of soluble fibre. The proportions of soluble and insoluble fibre in fruits and vegetables vary but they generally contain a substantially higher proportion of soluble NSP than wheat fibre, the major source of cereal fibre in the UK diet. Pulses (beans and peas) are generally high in soluble fibre. Many heat-processed starchy foods contain starch that resists digestion by human gut enzymes and thus probably acts like fibre in the intestine. Bread, cornflakes, boiled potatoes and boiled rice contain substantial amounts of this 'resistant starch' (reviewed by Berry, 1988).

Increased intakes of dietary fibre increase the volume of stools produced and reduce the transit time (the time it takes for ingested material to pass out in the faeces). The components of dietary fibre are fermented to a variable degree by intestinal bacteria (soluble components are generally the most readily fermentable). This fermentation leads to increased proliferation of intestinal bacteria and thus increases the bacterial mass in the stools. The fatty acids produced during fermentation also tend to acidify the colonic contents and may act as a stimulant to propulsion through the bowel. Intestinal gas is a by-product of this fermentation process. The unfermented components of fibre hold water and thus also increase the stool bulk and make the stools softer and easier to pass. The increased bulk and softness of stools, together with more direct effects on gut motility produced by the products of fermentation, combine to accelerate the passage of faeces through the colon (fibre/NSP reviewed by Halliday and Ashwell, 1991).

Some fibre-rich foods are:

- wholegrain breakfast cereals
- other wholegrain cereals foods (e.g. wholemeal bread, brown rice)
- fruit and vegetables, especially with their edible skins (e.g. baked potatoes)
- pulse vegetables (e.g. baked beans, kidney beans and lentils)
- dried fruit and nuts.

Bran should be used only if it has been medically prescribed and it must be introduced slowly. When introduced to a previously low fibre diet it may lead to stomach pains, diarrhoea and flatulence. In addition, it may reduce the absorption of calcium and iron by the body. It is vital that extra fluid is consumed if bran has been prescribed.

Diabetes mellitus

INTRODUCTION

Diabetes mellitus results from a relative or absolute lack of the pancreatic hormone insulin. Almost 5% of over 65s in the UK are recognised diabetics but the true prevalence may be more than double this (DH, 1991). In the severe, type I form, which usually develops during childhood, there is destruction of the insulin producing cells in the pancreas which results in an almost total failure of insulin supply. In the much more common and milder type II form of the disease, there is a progressive inadequacy of insulin production. This inadequacy seems to stem from a failure of the pancreas to be able to adequately compensate for a progressive decline in sensitivity to insulin in the target tissues. More insulin is needed to get the same effect and the diabetic seems unable to compensate adequately by producing the extra insulin. The 'western' diet and lifestyle seem to be triggers for this decline in insulin sensitivity; likely contributing factors are overweight, inactivity and a high fat/high energy diet (see Chapter 4). Diet is thus seen as an important aetiological factor for this type of diabetes.

Diabetics are divided clinically into those that require insulin replacement therapy (insulin-dependent diabetes mellitus, IDDM) and those who do not (non-insulin-dependent diabetes mellitus, NIDDM). All type I diabetics are insulin dependent and some type II diabetics may progress to the stage where they become dependent upon insulin or where effective management and sense of wellbeing requires the use of insulin.

Diet has historically been a key element in the management of diabetes. Around one-third of all diagnosed diabetics are treated with insulin and diet, around one-third are treated with oral antidiabetic drugs and diet, whilst the remainder are treated by diet alone.

DIAGNOSIS OF DIABETES

All diabetics have high blood glucose concentration and, as a consequence, they excrete glucose in their urine which also causes increased water loss, increased thirst and propensity to dehydration. A range of symptoms may cause sufferers to visit the general practitioner, for example:

- excessive thirst
- tiredness
- polyuria (passing lots of urine)
- blurred vision
- recurrent genitourinary tract infections.

The problems of rapid weight loss, excessive production of ketones and the associated, and potentially acutely life-threatening, acidotic coma are usually confined to type I diabetics who will make up only a tiny proportion of elderly diabetics. Indeed, in older patients, symptoms may be so mild that they remain unrecognised for many years. Ketosis is uncommon in elderly diabetics and they are usually overweight rather than underweight. Many older diabetics are diagnosed at routine health checks when a sample of urine is tested; the urine contains glucose and a subsequent blood test records a raised blood glucose.

A glucose tolerance test (GTT) can be used to confirm the diagnosis; after an overnight fast the patient is given an oral glucose load and blood glucose concentration is recorded at thirty minute intervals for 2–3 hours. In a healthy young subject, blood glucose will rise from around 4–5 mmol/l up to 7–8 mmol/l in response to the oral load but will return to the resting level within 2–3 hours. In diabetics, the resting level may be higher and the blood glucose will rise higher and stay elevated for an extended period. The magnitude of this abnormal glucose tolerance determines whether the patient is classified as 'frankly diabetic' or 'impaired glucose tolerance' (i.e. prediabetic or borderline diabetic).

EVOLVING AIMS AND STRATEGIES IN THE DIETARY MANAGEMENT OF DIABETES

The symptoms of diabetes suggest carbohydrate intolerance and so severe restriction of dietary carbohydrate, and almost total exclusion of dietary sugar, have been the rule for diabetic diets for most of this century. Prior to the 1970s most diabetic diets would have contained no more than 40% of the calories as carbohydrates and in many cases much less than this; such diets were inevitably high in fat (Keen and Thomas, 1988). The historical priority of diabetic therapy has been to alleviate the immediate symptoms of the disease which in IDDM are acutely life-threatening.

In older diabetics the disease is not usually acutely life-threatening but, in addition to the acute symptoms, diabetics of both types have a greatly increased risk of suffering from a range of long-term secondary complications that increase their morbidity and reduce life expectancy, for example:

- cardiovascular diseases that are precipitated by atherosclerosis
- progressive loss of renal function (diabetic nephropathy)
- progressive damage to the retina (diabetic retinopathy)
- cataract
- degeneration of peripheral nerves with loss of sensation (peripheral neuropathy)
- gangrene (particularly in the feet and legs) which may lead to amputation.

In some elderly patients these secondary complications of diabetes may be the presenting symptoms because the acute symptoms are so mild. A major objective of modern diabetic therapy is to reduce the toll of these longterm complications of diabetes.

Two major considerations seem to be important in this respect. The high rate of cardiovascular disease seen in 'western' diabetics does not seem to be an inevitable consequence of diabetes. Japanese and black East African diabetics have been relatively free of cardiovascular disease unlike either Japanese American or black American diabetics (Keen and Thomas, 1988). A high fat diet is widely accepted to be a risk factor for cardiovascular diseases and so the traditional (pre-1980), very high fat diet and consequent hyperlipidaemia of diabetics has almost certainly been a factor in their propensity to cardiovascular disease.

Diabetics also suffer from a range of conditions that are attributed to degenerative changes in their microvasculature (i.e. capillaries). These changes in the microvasculature are probably responsible for the diabetic retinopathy that causes many diabetics to go blind and also for the high levels of renal disease seen in diabetics. Changes in the capillaries of diabetics are thought to stem from a chemical change in their membrane proteins brought about by their continued exposure to high glucose levels. A similar mechanism is probably responsible for the development of cataract and the degeneration of peripheral nerves and gangrene often seen in older diabetics.

Modern diabetic management of the elderly seeks to reduce these longer term complications by:

• achieving and maintaining a normal body weight
• minimising hyperlipidaemia and hyperglycaemia.

Good glycaemic control is a priority for diabetic management. The results of the Diabetes Control and Complications Trial (DCCT, 1993) showed convincing evidence that better control reduced the risk of developing the complications of diabetes such as nephropathy, retinopathy and neuropathy. Although this study was conducted in younger, insulin-dependent diabetics it seems likely that the general conclusions also apply to older non-insulin-dependent diabetics. There is now greatly increased priority attached to normalisation of the blood lipid levels of diabetics because of the mass of evidence implicating hyperlipidaemia as a major cause of atherosclerosis; this should reduce the toll from cardiovascular diseases in older diabetics.

THE MODERN DIABETIC DIET – AN OVERVIEW

In order to achieve the above goals, the diet recommended for diabetics has changed very considerably over the past 20 years and is almost the opposite of that previously recommended. From a high fat, low carbohydrate, very low sugar diet to a high carbohydrate, moderate sugar, moderate fat diet. The modern recommended diabetic diet has more than half of the calories from carbohydrate with the emphasis on unrefined foods high in complex carbohydrate and fibre. It has moderate levels of fat and saturated fat and even the very strict avoidance of sugar has been relaxed, provided that it is a component of a meal. The general avoidance of isolated sugary foods (except for hypoglycaemic emergency in IDDM) is still recommended.   A diet considered ideal for diabetics with NIDDM is very similar to that recommended for the population as a whole; it should have the following overall composition:

- **carbohydrate** 50–55% of the total dietary energy intake, the majority from complex sources (i.e. foods that are also naturally rich in dietary fibre or hydrolysis-resistant starch)
- **fat** 30–35% of total dietary energy intake with a maximum of 10% from saturated fats
- **protein** 10–15% of total dietary energy intake.

BODY WEIGHT CONTROL

There is a strong correlation between obesity and risk of NIDDM. Normalisation of body weight and regulation of caloric intake to match expenditure may in some cases completely alleviate the symptoms of NIDDM. Increases in activity are therefore likely to be of particular benefit for overweight diabetics. A low fat and low sugar diet that is high in complex carbohydrate is the current basis of orthodox reducing diets and so it is perhaps only in overall energy level that the diet of the overweight and normal weight diabetic should differ. Energy-free, artificial sweeteners such as aspartame and saccharin may be useful in diabetic management, particularly the use of low calorie soft drinks. Many of the special 'diabetic foods' have sorbitol or fructose as their sweetening agent and although these are absorbed more slowly than glucose they have similar energy contents to the equivalent standard foods. These diabetic foods are often expensive and they are not a necessary or even desirable component of diabetic diets, unless they are also low in calories.

RATIONALE FOR INCREASING STARCH AND FIBRE INTAKES

Diabetic diets were traditionally low in carbohydrate and high in fat. Keen and Thomas (1988) suggest that much of the success of these traditional low carbohydrate diabetic diets may have been due to their regulation of energy intake rather than carbohydrate restriction *per se*. They argue that provided the diabetic is in energy balance, short term diabetic control is not really affected by the proportion of calories from fat or carbohydrate. A raised carbohydrate intake increases peripheral sensitivity to insulin and thus does not increase the need for insulin. This adaptation cannot, of course, occur in the absence of insulin and so carbohydrate does have adverse effects in untreated IDDM thus explaining the past assumption that carbohydrate was inevitably bad for all diabetics.

Simpson (1981) concluded that an increase in the proportion of energy from carbohydrate, together with an increase in dietary fibre, has a generally favourable effect upon blood glucose control in both types of diabetes. The reduction in fat content that is a consequence of raising the carbohydrate content of diabetic diets, reduces blood lipid levels and should contribute to a reduction in atherosclerosis.

The effects of fibre (non-starch polysaccharide, NSP) in improving glucose tolerance are well documented (see Halliday and Ashwell, 1991). Increases in dietary fibre have been recommended for the population as a whole and are particularly recommended for diabetics for the following reasons.

- Increased fibre content of foods slows down the rate of glucose absorption from the gut and thus reduces the post prandial peak concentrations of glucose and insulin in blood. This effect is attributed primarily to the soluble components of NSP and it is thought to be due to delayed stomach emptying and the mechanical effect of the viscous NSP components in reducing the contact of dissolved glucose with the absorptive surface of the intestinal epithelium.
- Fibre may have beneficial effects on blood lipids. This may be because it promotes the faecal loss of biliary cholesterol and reduces absorption and reabsorption of cholesterol from the gut.
- High fibre diets are inevitably of low energy density (energy per gram of food) this should assist in weight control. Blundell and Burley (1987) review evidence that NSP may also have a satiating effect. It is suggested that this might be because high NSP foods slow eating speed, slow gastric emptying and contribute to feelings of fullness, and because they slow down the absorption of nutrients reducing the insulin response to absorbed nutrients. A large insulin response to absorbed nutrients may cause blood glucose concentration to fall below resting levels (the rebound effect), triggering feelings of hunger.

BENEFITS OF REDUCED FAT IN THE DIABETIC DIET

A reduction in fat and saturated fat intake would be desirable for NIDDM diabetics on several grounds, as follows.

- It should lead to a reduction in plasma lipid levels and thus reduce susceptibility to atherosclerosis.
- It would inevitably decrease the energy density of the diet as fat yields more than twice as many calories per gram as the other major sources of dietary energy.
- Fat may be less satiating than carbohydrate, over and above any effect upon energy density (therefore perhaps more fattening).
- Low fat diets are more likely to be high in fibre and starch.

CONCLUSION

NIDDM is a common, chronic condition for many older people. Dietary treatment is indicated at all ages; in many cases this is effective in alleviating symptoms and maintaining normal blood glucose levels. In some cases oral hypoglycaemic drugs are used in combination with a dietary prescription and, less frequently in elderly patients, insulin injections may be required for effective management. The basic prescription is a reduced fat, reduced sugar, high carbohydrate and high fibre diet, similar to that recommended for the general adult population.

A gradual loss of weight in obese, diabetic patients is desirable and this loss may lead to a substantial reduction in symptoms. Where practical and acceptable, an increased level of physical activity, such as walking, should be an important component of the weight loss strategy.

Obesity

WHO SHOULD BE TREATED?

According to a large survey of English adults (White *et al.*, 1993) about 10% of men over 65 and 17% of elderly women are classified as obese with a body mass index of greater than 30. A further 40–45% of elderly people are overweight with a BMI between 25 and 30. The prevalence of obesity declines with age amongst elderly people, falling from 14% in 65–74-year-old men to 7% in those aged over 75 years; corresponding figures for women are 19% and 16% respectively.

In young and middle-aged adults, there is a very substantial body of evidence that being overweight and particularly being obese is associated with increased morbidity and mortality from a large number of causes (see Chapter 4). In older adults, obesity may have a negative impact upon mobility and immobility leads to a decline in physical and mental wellbeing. On the other hand, evidence has been discussed in Chapters 4 and 5 that the predictive relationship between overweight/obesity and subsequent mortality changes with age; from being a predictor of higher mortality risk amongst young and middle-aged people (especially men) to being a predictor of lower mortality risk in very elderly people. There could be several explanations for this latter observation and it certainly does not mean that helping any elderly, obese person to lose weight will inevitably hasten their demise nor that there should be no attempts to treat obesity in any elderly person. It does suggest that a degree of caution and selectivity should be exercised in the treatment of obesity and more especially overweight in the elderly. There seems to be little hard information upon which to base any strict criteria about when to treat obesity in the elderly. However, the following factors would be expected to influence that clinical judgement.

- **The degree of morbidity or incapacity that is attributable to the obesity or the degree to which obesity might exacerbate other medical conditions.** In the previous section, the role of obesity in precipitating diabetes in susceptible elderly people was discussed; in this case weight loss often ameliorates the symptoms of the diabetes. Other examples of morbidities associated with obesity would be reduced mobility, including any exacerbating effects on osteoarthritis, and severe hypertension. In several other medical conditions, the symptoms might be exacerbated by obesity (e.g. heart failure and chronic bronchitis).
- **The degree of overweight/obesity and the age of the patient.** The threshold at which a decision to intervene to reduce body weight might be expected to increase with age unless there are additional grounds for intervention such as those discussed above. One might well conclude that specific intervention with the overweight elderly should be restricted to those cases where there are other medical indications for weight loss or where the patient is personally motivated to lose weight to enhance their own self-esteem.

- **The effect that dietary restriction would have on nutrient adequacy,** especially with an ill and/or bedridden elderly person. Such patients may not be eating enough to achieve dietary adequacy and restricting intake may compound the problem.
- **The adverse effect that dietary restriction may have upon the total quality of life of the elderly person.**

STRATEGIES FOR THE TREATMENT OF OBESITY

The basic elements of conventional weight reduction regimens are:

- an attempt to increase energy expenditure by encouraging a moderate and gradual increase in physical activity. This advice would probably be beneficial to the vast majority of healthy elderly people irrespective of whether or not they are overweight.
- a modification of the diet structure, moving closer to the 'ideals' suggested by the *Food Guide Pyramid* and *Food Guide Plate* described in Chapter 2 or the CWT (1995) standards for community meals and meals in residential homes given in Chapter 7; an increase in the proportion of energy obtained from cereals, fruits and vegetables with reduced consumption of sugary and fatty foods (i.e. a high carbohydrate, high fibre, reduced fat and low sugar diet). Once again this advice could non-controversially be given to the vast majority of healthy elderly people.
- a specific attempt to reduce calorie intake to less than expenditure (i.e. to induce negative energy balance). It is in this third aspect, the prescription of a specific, calorie reduced diet, that the greater selectivity discussed previously needs to be applied. If the first two measures were adopted, then, in the long-term, they alone might be expected to lead to moderation of overweight and obesity in a substantial proportion of elderly people without any specific attempts to restrain calorie intake.

ACHIEVING WEIGHT LOSS

It is important to set realistic goals for weight loss; 0.25–0.50 kg/week is a reasonable target. A slow, steady loss is more likely to be effective in the longer term than rapid weight losses brought about by short term 'crash diets'. The areas for modification of the existing diet and eating pattern need to be identified and accepted by the client. The client must be persuaded that the new 'healthy eating' is for life and not a short-term measure that will lead to rapid weight loss whence they can return to their previous habits. If non-hunger cues like boredom, loneliness or depression cause an individual to overeat then dealing with these problems may be more effective than trying to ensure adherence to a strict dietary prescription.

Some hints for weight loss that may be useful to older people:

- eat three regular meals a day and avoid sweet snacks between meals
- eat slowly and carefully, concentrating on what you are doing; switch off the television
- avoid fried food: grill, poach, boil and bake instead

- increase the quantity of fruit and vegetables consumed
- reduce the fat content by removing visible fat from meat and by eating less butter and margarine
- change to semi-skimmed milk
- cut out sweets, sugar in tea/coffee and other visible sources of sugar; make use of artificial sweeteners if required
- drink sugar-free soft drinks
- eat wholemeal bread and wholegrain cereals
- do not feel guilty after an occasional lapse
- moderate the use of alcohol.

PRACTICAL CONSIDERATIONS

- Many old people have a very limited budget. Switching to a diet which makes more use of cereals and vegetables should in theory reduce over-all food costs. However, if the older person tries to maintain a diet as close to their original diet as possible (e.g. by choosing reduced fat and sugar versions of their normal foods) then this 'least change' diet is likely to involve substantial extra expenditure (Groom, 1993). Budgeting consider-ations must be taken into account when giving dietary advice to older people.
- Where an elderly person is inactive, energy expenditure may be very low. It is essential that the regulated amount of food provided for in any dietary prescription fulfils all of the client's nutrient needs.
- A slow steady loss of weight should be the goal with moderate physical activity wherever possible.
- Acutely ill people should generally not commence a weight reducing regime. They are likely to lose lean body mass rather than body fat and become more deficient in a range of vitamins and minerals. Under these circumstances, the supply of essential nutrients is the overriding priority.
- Some people enjoy the support of others when trying to lose weight. Slimming clubs can be a social boost as well as an opportunity to gain use-ful information and support.

Hyperlipidaemia

Hyperlipidaemia means a high blood lipid content. There are several types of hyperlipidaemia. Some of these are congenital disorders and are associated with high rates of mortality prior to old age; these will, therefore, be exclud-ed from this discussion on treatment of hyperlipidaemia in the elderly. Fats/lipids are insoluble in water so their transport in plasma requires that they be associated with protein carriers and transported as lipid/protein aggregates or lipoproteins. The principal lipoproteins in plasma are:

- chylomicrons
- very low density lipoproteins – VLDL
- low density lipoproteins – LDL
- high density lipoproteins – HDL.

Chylomicrons are the form in which ingested fat is transported to the liver and tissues after its absorption from the intestine. They are normally absent from fasting blood and severe elevation of chylomicron levels is usually associated with a rare congenital defect; it is not usually a problem of the elderly. The principal lipoproteins in fasting blood are VLDL, LDL and HDL.

HYPERTRIGLYCERIDAEMIA

VLDL is rich in triglyceride so measures of fasting blood triglycerides are taken to indicate the amount of VLDL. The normal function of VLDL is to transport endogenously produced triglycerides from their site of synthesis (the liver) to their sites of storage (adipose tissue) or of use as an energy source. Raised VLDL is associated with obesity, glucose intolerance and high alcohol consumption. Hyperlipidaemia that is characterised solely by a raised VLDL (raised blood triglycerides) is designated as hyperlipidaemia type IV. This condition is associated with increased risk of cardiovascular disease but there is some debate as to whether raised triglyceride levels are independently linked to cardiovascular disease after allowing for the associated obesity, glucose intolerance (diabetes) and/or alcohol abuse. Treatment of this condition is geared towards addressing the underlying cause, i.e. normalising body weight in overweight subjects, treating the diabetes in those with seriously impaired glucose tolerance and moderating alcohol use. Consumption of oily fish (e.g. herring, mackerel, trout and salmon) or fish oil capsules has a lowering effect on blood triglyceride levels. Reduced consumption of sugars may also be used in this condition.

HYPERCHOLESTERAEMIA (SEE ALSO 'SERUM CHOLESTEROL' IN CHAPTER 4)

Cholesterol is a normal and essential component of cell membranes and it is also the starting point for the synthesis of the steroid hormones in the adrenal glands and gonads. LDL is the major cholesterol-containing fraction in the plasma (LDL contains around two-thirds of the plasma cholesterol) and thus measures of serum cholesterol are taken to indicate the LDL. LDL acts as an external source of cholesterol for cells unable to synthesise sufficient for use in membranes or as a precursor for steroid hormone synthesis. HDL is the smaller component of the total plasma cholesterol and HDL serves to transport excess cholesterol from tissues back to the liver.

Epidemiological evidence and evidence from people with familial hypercholesteraemia (hyperlipidaemia type IIa) suggest that high plasma LDL cholesterol concentrations are associated with an increased risk of coronary heart disease and that the association is probably causative. Many people (especially men) with congenitally high LDL levels die from premature heart disease. High HDL cholesterol concentrations seem to be protective against coronary heart disease and the LDL to HDL ratio may be a better predictor of coronary heart disease risk than LDL concentration alone (Oliver, 1981).

In young and middle-aged people, an elevated plasma cholesterol concentration is generally accepted to be causally associated with an increased risk of coronary heart disease and, at least in men in these age groups, is associated with increased total mortality. The relationship between plasma cholesterol, heart disease and total mortality risk is much less clear in the elderly and also in women (discussed at length in Chapter 4).

WHEN SHOULD HYPERCHOLESTERAEMIA BE TREATED IN THE ELDERLY?

The answer to this question is clearly a matter of clinical judgement that will hopefully be based upon a holistic assessment of the pros and cons of treatment for each individual patient.

Dunnigan (1993) and Smith et al. (1993) discuss this problem and both imply that the evidence upon which to base such a decision is currently incomplete and likely to remain so for the foreseeable future. Smith et al. specifically suggest the need for trials that seek to clarify the level of risk of coronary heart disease due to hypercholesteraemia, at which treatment is of net benefit to patients.

It has been suggested that 5.2 mmol/l is the top of the optimal range for plasma cholesterol concentration, but over 80% of elderly British men and 95% of elderly women have values in excess of this (White et al., 1993). It has further been suggested that 7.8 mmol/l is the point at which plasma cholesterol should be designated as severely elevated or frankly hypercholesteraemic. Almost a quarter of elderly British women and 2% of elderly men would be hypercholesteraemic by this definition. In the current dietary and nutritional survey of the UK elderly population, a figure of 8 mmol/l has been adopted as the cut-off point for hypercholesteraemia (Hughes, 1995). Evidence from intervention trials suggests that cholesterol lowering interventions tend only to yield measurable holistic benefits in patients who have the highest risk of dying of coronary heart disease, e.g. patients with frank hypercholesteraemia and/or existing coronary heart disease. In lower risk patients, intervention, especially intervention that includes the use of cholesterol-lowering drugs, may actually increase total mortality. Current evidence, therefore suggests caution in the use of specific cholesterol-lowering interventions in elderly people and that the criteria for treatment should be increasingly demanding as the level of intervention increases, i.e. most discriminating where cholesterol-lowering drugs are used.

LEVELS OF INTERVENTION FOR HYPERCHOLESTERAEMIA

General risk factor reduction. Hypercholesteraemia is one of a number of risk factors for coronary heart disease. Some are unalterable (e.g. sex and genetic make-up) but several others are alterable, for example:

- smoking
- inactivity
- hypertension
- obesity
- stress.

The impact of these risk factors, including hypercholesteraemia, is cumulative. Reduced tobacco usage, increased activity, weight control and control of blood pressure will reduce risk of coronary heart disease in their own right. They will also produce other health benefits and complement any lowering of plasma cholesterol concentration.

General dietary guidelines. The general dietary guidelines for the population (discussed specifically in Chapter 2) would be expected to lead to some reduction in plasma cholesterol as well as being expected to yield several other health benefits. This implies moderation of dietary fat (to around 35% of food energy) and saturated fat (15%) with a corresponding increase in consumption of starch and non-starch polysaccharide (fibre); reduced consumption of fats and oils, fatty meats, dairy fats and increased consumption of cereals, fruits and vegetables.

A specifically cholesterol-lowering diet. This diet would involve more severe limitation on fat (no more than 30% of food energy) and saturated fat (less than 10% of food energy). There would be increased emphasis on reducing the saturation of the fat that was permitted (e.g. by emphasising the use of highly polyunsaturated or highly monounsaturated cooking and spreading fats). There might also be some attempt to specifically reduce the amount of dietary cholesterol. Dietary cholesterol would tend to fall as saturated fat intake fell but in addition, some low to moderate fat foods are high in cholesterol and might be restricted (e.g. prawns and other shellfish, eggs and liver).

Fatty fish and fish oil supplements. It has already been suggested that fish oils (from fatty fish or concentrated supplements) have a lowering effect on plasma triglycerides. They may also have a small cholesterol-lowering effect. More significantly for patients at high risk of coronary thrombosis, fish oils may reduce the coagulability of blood; in experimental studies large doses of fish oils have been found to reduce blood clotting and to extend the bleeding time (e.g. Sanders, 1985). Fish oils also seem to have an anti-inflammatory effect and this may be important in reducing the post infarction inflammatory damage to the heart after a heart attack. This anti-inflammatory effect may also explain the suggested benefits on inflammatory diseases like arthritis and eczema. In a controlled, secondary intervention trial of fish oils on patients who had previously suffered a myocardial infarction, fish oils significantly reduced both cardiovascular and total mortality whereas the other treatments (low fat diets or increased cereal fibre) did not (Burr *et al.*, 1991). In this trial, the fish oil patients did not have significantly fewer re-infarcts but these new infarcts were less likely to be fatal – consistent with this suggestion of reduced post-infarct inflammatory damage.

Current evidence seems to support the case for specifically recommending increases in fatty fish consumption or even the use of fish oil supplements in those with established coronary heart disease and/or some types of hyperlipidaemia. The overall evidence at present seems consistent with the recommendation that fish and fatty fish be included in healthful and diverse diets for those who like fish and have no cultural objections to consuming fish. There is no compelling evidence to warrant recommending universal consumption of fish oil supplements or even consumption of fatty fish on purely therapeutic grounds. For persons at high and immediate risk of coronary thrombosis, reduced tendency for blood to clot may be considered a beneficial effect but would it be necessarily good for everyone? (e.g. those with some existing defect in the clotting system or those at high risk of cerebral haemorrhage). A short, referenced and non-specialist review of fish oils may be found in Webb (1995). Small doses of aspirin have a similar antithrombotic effect to that described for fish oils.

Use of cholesterol-lowering drugs. There is a range of drugs that exert a cholesterol-lowering effect; detailed discussion of their use and mode of action is beyond the scope of this book. Evidence from several intervention trials (e.g. Smith, 1993) suggests that they should be used cautiously. When used on persons not at high risk of coronary heart disease excess mortality/morbidity associated with side-effects of the drug may cancel out or even exceed any benefits of reduced plasma cholesterol and consequent reduced risk of coronary heart disease.

Some of these agents act by binding or chelating cholesterol in the gut and so preventing the normal re-absorption and recycling of bile acid cholesterol (enterohepatic recycling). This increases the faecal losses of cholesterol but the drugs also tend to inhibit the absorption of fat soluble vitamins. The soluble fraction of dietary fibre (soluble NSP) may exert a small cholesterol lowering effect by a similar mechanism. A number of controlled studies have indicated that consumption of relatively large quantities of oats, which are rich in soluble NSP, can have a significant cholesterol-lowering effect in subjects with either elevated or normal cholesterol levels. Other cholesterol-lowering agents act by inhibiting key enzymes on the pathway of cholesterol synthesis and thus they reduce cholesterol production. Yet others accelerate the clearance of LDL from the plasma.

Dementia

INTRODUCTION

Psychogeriatric conditions can be classified as organic or functional. Organic conditions involve morphological changes in the brain which can, for example, can be identified at autopsy (e.g. Alzheimer's disease, Parkinson's disease, Huntingdon's Chorea and Creutzfeld-Jacob disease). The functional psychiatric diseases are those where there is no such obvious morphological change in the brain and would include depression, paranoia, schizophrenia, psychoses and neuroses.

The functional disorders affect all age groups and account for most mental illness in younger adults. The prevalence of clinical depression amongst elderly people in the UK has been estimated at between 5% and 20%. In the free-living elderly the prevalence is higher in those not currently married and those living alone; it may well be higher still amongst those living in some residential homes. There is considerable evidence that functional mental illnesses, particularly depressive illnesses, can have very marked effects upon food intake but this topic will not be discussed in this book. We will concentrate upon those conditions that are specifically associated with the elderly, that is dementia. As the incidence of dementia increases sharply with age amongst the elderly and as the very elderly (over 85 years) is a very rapidly growing proportion of the population it would seem that there are inevitably going to be rapid increases in the numbers of people suffering from dementia in the coming decades.

INCIDENCE OF DEMENTIA

The prevalence of dementia and the organic diseases increases with age. The prevalence of dementia in all people aged over 65 years in the UK has been variously estimated at between 5% and 7% but with a marked tendency to rise with age and more than 20% of those over 75 years may be affected. In persons aged 65–74 years dementia accounts for about 18% of all admissions to mental hospitals but this rises to well over 40% of admissions in those aged over 85 years. Alzheimer's disease is the most prevalent form of dementia and it has been suggested that the incidence may be 20 times higher in those aged 80 years as compared to those aged 60 years. In a survey of 12 local authority residential homes for the elderly, one-third of residents had severe dementia and a further third had mild to moderate dementia; note that these were not nursing homes but homes that only accepted patients able to perform certain task of everyday living independently (DH, 1991). After heart disease, cancer and stroke, Alzheimer's disease is the fourth leading cause of death in the developed world (Duff and Hardy, 1995).

ALZHEIMER'S DISEASE

Alzheimer's disease is a progressive disorder which can be divided into three stages. In the first stage there is loss of memory, partial disorientation and lack of spontaneous emotional response. The second stage is characterised by an inability to identify familiar sights, sounds or smells. The person may not recognise family members or familiar settings, food or eating utensils; erratic non-purposeful movements may begin at this stage. In the third stage, seizures develop, speech is lost and the patient is indifferent to his or her environment. Non-purposeful movements may become more intense. The sufferer usually has little interest in food and food is often played with rather than eaten. As the disease progresses through the final stage the patient might show signs of compulsive eating or alternatively refuse to eat or try to eat objects that are inedible.

Diagnosis of Alzheimer's disease is made by clinical examination although this may not be conclusive as the signs and symptoms are common to other forms of dementia. The second most common cause of irreversible dementia is multi-infarct dementia which is a result of many small strokes in the brain. A small number of dementia cases may be the result of such conditions as alcoholism, cerebral tumours, thyroid disease and vitamin B_{12} deficiency.

NUTRITION AND DEMENTIA

There has been a limited amount of work on the nutritional intakes of dementia patients but this work suggests that intakes are often very low. Many of these patients are very underweight, particularly in the later stages of the disease. It has been suggested that these patients may be hypermetabolic and that high energy requirements may be a cause of weight loss. However, Prentice *et al.* (1989) measured total energy expenditure (using the doubly-labelled-water method) together with food and fluid intakes in a group of elderly dementia patients with deteriorating nutritional status. They were able to show convincingly that these patients actually had relatively low metabolic rates, low total energy expenditures and that the cause of their undernutrition was undoubtedly inadequate food intake. In an unpublished study, one of the authors (JC) analysed the energy and nutrient contents of menus offered to psychogeriatric (largely dementia) patients in long stay Bristol hospitals. The menus provided an inadequate amount of energy, even allowing for unrecorded snacks.

The nutritional and eating problems of dementia patients change as the disease progresses. In the early phase there may be problems like forgetting to eat, eating food which is too hot, eating non-foods, gorging, eating spoilt foods, difficulties in shopping and preparing food. There is often a change in food choice, with preference towards sweet and salty foods and sometimes bizarre food choices. Some patients may have difficulty in feeding themselves or a reduced ability to co-ordinate chewing, swallowing and facial movements. During the second phase there is an increase in activity with the patient becoming agitated. Food can be hoarded in the mouth rather than swallowed and the ability to use cutlery properly is diminished. In the final phase, food is often not recognised and patients may refuse to open their

Table 8.2 Some practical steps to improve the food intake of demented patients. Source: after Thomas (1994)

Minimise distractions such as the television at mealtimes.
Portion sizes should be appropriate to the individual.
Modified utensils may help if the patient has difficulty using normal ones.
Some patients eat better alone than in groups.
Avoid mixed textures of foods.
Do not fill glasses and cups to the top but allow room for shaking as a person moves the glass or cup to their mouth.
Present only one course at a time.
An encouraging, friendly atmosphere and positive approach to mealtimes is important. A relaxed atmosphere with minimal distractions may help improve the food intake.

mouths or turn away when food is offered. The patient is unable to ask for food or drink and the patient may have difficulty swallowing and initiating movements to open their mouth or chew. Table 8.2 shows some practical steps that may improve the food intake and help maintain the nutritional status of dementia patients.

MALNUTRITION AS A CAUSE OF NEUROLOGICAL SYMPTOMS IN THE ELDERLY

Some nutritional deficiencies are known to give rise to severe neurological symptoms; in some cases the symptoms can be alleviated by correction of the nutrient deficit. For example:

- thiamine deficiency can give rise to Wernicke's encephalopathy (often associated with alcoholism in industrialised countries) and mild deficiency may be a factor in acute confusional states in the elderly (COMA, 1992)
- dementia is one of the symptoms of pellagra (niacin deficiency)
- dehydration can cause an acute confusional state
- deficiencies of vitamin B_{12} and folate may give rise to depression and mild cognitive impairment (COMA, 1992).

Morgan and Schorah (1986) tried to assess the importance of nutritional disorders in causing and aggravating psychogeriatric problems. They concluded that although severe nutrient deficiency may undoubtedly be a cause of neurological symptoms, the number of elderly patients affected is probably small. They further concluded that less severe deficiencies probably only make a marginal contribution to psychogeriatric problems in a minority of patients.

References

Ajzen, I. and Fishbein, M. 1980 *Understanding attitudes and predicting social behaviour.* Engelwood Cliffs, New Jersey: Prentice-Hall.

Allied Dunbar National Fitness Survey. 1992 *A report on activity patterns and fitness levels.* London: Sports Council.

Ashwell, M. 1992 The BNF Task Force Report on unsaturated fatty acids. *British Nutrition Foundation Nutrition Bulletin* 17, 160-163.

Ashwell, M. 1993 Trans in transition. *British Nutrition Foundation Nutrition Bulletin* 18, 150–153.

Bassey, E.J. 1985 Benefits of exercise in the elderly. In: *Recent advances in geriatric medicine 3* Ed Issago, B. Edinburgh: Churchill Livingstone.

Bastow, M.D., Rawlings, J. and Allison, S.P. 1983 Benefits of supplementary tube feeding after fractured neck of femur; a randomised controlled trial. *British Medical Journal* 287, 1589–1592.

Bebbington, A.C. 1988 The expectation of life without disability in England and Wales. *Social Science and Medicine* 27, 321–326.

Becker, M.H. (ed) 1984 *The health belief model and personal health behaviour.* Thorofare, New Jersey: Charles B. Slack.

Bennett, K. and Morgan, K. 1992 Activity and morale in later life: preliminary analyses from the Nottingham Longitudinal Study of Activity and Ageing. In: *Nutrition and physical activity.* ed. Norgan, N.G. Cambridge: Cambridge University Press. pp. 129–142.

Berry, C.S. 1988 Resistant starch – a controversial component of dietary fibre. *British Nutrition Foundation Nutrition Bulletin* 13, 141–152.

Bistrian, B.R., Blackburn, G.L., Hallowell, E. and Heddle, R. 1974 Protein status of general surgical patients. *Journal of the American Medical Association* 230, 858–860.

Blair, S.N., Kohl, H.W., Paffenbarger, R.S., Clark, D.G., Cooper, K.H. and Gibbons, L.W. 1989 Physical fitness and all cause mortality. A prospective study of healthy men and women. *Journal of the American Medical Association* 262, 2395–2401.

Blundell, J.E. and Burley, V.J. 1987 Satiation, satiety and the action of dietary fibre on food intake. *International Journal of Obesity* 11 supp 1, 9–25.

Brown, D.R. 1992 Physical activity, ageing, and psychological well-being: an overview of the research. *Canadian Journal of Sport Science* 17(3), 185–193.

Brown, K. 1991 Improving Intakes. *Nursing Times* 87, 64–67

Brown, K. and Seabrook, N. 1992 Effect of nutrition on recovery after fractured femur. *Medical Audit News* 2(1), 10–12.

Burr, M.L. 1985. The nutritional state of the elderly: demographic and epidemiologic considerations. In: *Nutrition, immunity and illness in the elderly.* Chandra, R.K. ed. New York: Pergamon Press. pp. 7–18.

Burr, M.L., Fehily, A.M., Gilbert, J.F., Rogers, S., Holliday, R.M., Sweetnam, P.M., Elwood, P.C. and Deadman, N.M. 1991 Effects of changes in fat, fish and fibre intakes on death and myocardial infarction: Diet and reinfarction trial (DART). *Lancet* ii, 757–761.

Burr, M.L. and Phillips, K.M. 1984 Anthropometric norms in the elderly. *British Journal of Nutrition* 51, 165–169.

Campbell, A.J., Spears, G.F.S., Brown, J.S., Busby, W.J. and Borrie, M.J. 1990 Anthropometric measurements as predictors of mortality in a community aged 70 years and over. *Age and Ageing* 19, 131–135.

Cataldo, C.B., DeBruyne, L.K. and Whitney, E.R. 1995 *Nutrition and diet therapy* 4th edn. St. Paul, MN: West Publishing Company.

Caughey, P., Seaman, C., Parry, D., Farquar, D. and McNennan, W.J. 1994 Nutrition of old people in sheltered housing. *Journal of Human Nutrition and Dietetics* 7, 263–268.

Chandra, R.K. 1985 Nutrition-immunity-infection interactions in old age. In: *Nutrition, immunity and illness in the elderly.* Chandra, R.K. ed. New York: Pergamon Press. pp. 87–96.

Chandra, R.K. 1992 Effect of vitamin and trace-element supplementation on immune responses and infection in elderly subjects. *Lancet* 340, 1124–1126.

Chandra, R.K. 1993 Nutrition and the immune system. *Proceedings of the Nutrition Society* 52, 77–84.

Chapuy, M.C., Arlot, M.E., Delmas, P.D. and Meunier, P.J. 1994 Effects of calcium and cholecalciferol treatment for three years on hip fractures in elderly women. *British Medical Journal* 308, 1081–1082.

Chow, R., Harrison, J.E. and Notarius, C. 1987 Effect of two randomised exercise programmes on bone mass of healthy postmenopausal women. *British Medical Journal* 295, 1441–1444.

COMA 1991 Committee on Medical Aspects of Food Policy. *Dietary reference values for food energy and nutrients for the United Kingdom.* Report on health and social subjects No. 41. London: HMSO.

COMA 1992 Committee on Medical Aspects of Food Policy. *The nutrition of elderly people.* Report on health and social subjects no. 43. London: HMSO.

Crimmins, E.M., Saito, Y. and Ingegneri, D. 1989 Changes in life expectancy and disability-free life expectancy in the United States. *Population and Development Review* 15, 235–267.

Crowther, S. 1989 Eating well. *Geriatric Nursing and Home Care* Feb. 1989, 10–11.

CSO 1992 Central Statistical Office Expenditure Survey. *Family Spending 1991.* London: HMSO.

CSO 1993 Central Statistical Office Expenditure Survey. *Family Spending 1992.* London: HMSO.

Cummings, S.R., Kelsey, J.L., Nevitt, M.C. and O'Dowd, K.J. 1985 Epidemiology of osteoporosis and osteoporotic fractures. *Epidemiologic Reviews* 7, 178–208.

CWT 1995 The Caroline Walker Trust *Eating well for older people.* London: The Caroline Walker Trust

Davies, J. and Dickerson, J.W.T. 1991 *Nutrient content of food portions.* Cambridge: Royal Society of Chemistry.

Davies, L. 1988 Practical nutrition for the elderly. *Nutrition Reviews* 46(2), 83–87.

Davies, L. and Holdsworth, M. D. 1979 A technique for assessing nutritional "at risk" factors in residential homes for the elderly. *Journal of Human Nutrition* 33, 165–169.

Davies, L. and Knutson, K.C. 1991 Warning signals for malnutrition in the elderly. *Journal of the American Dietetic Association* 91 (ii), 1413–1417.

Davies, L. and Scotts, H. 1994 The Cost of Care. *Health Service Journal* 104, 31.

DCCT, The Diabetes Control and Complications Trial Research Group 1993 The effect of intensive treatment of diabetes on the development and progression of long term complications in insulin-dependent diabetes mellitus. *New England Journal of Medicine* 329, 977–86.

Debenham, K. 1992 Nutrition for specific disease conditions. In: *Nutrition and the consumer*. ed. Walker, A.F. and Rolls, B.A. London: Elsevier Applied Science. pp. 249–270.

Delmi, M., Rapin, C-H., Delmas, P.D., Vasey, H. and Bonjour, J-P. 1990 Dietary supplementation in elderly patients with fractured neck of the femur. *Lancet* 335, 1013–1016.

DH 1991 Department of Health. *On the state of the public health* 1990. London: HMSO.

DH 1992a Department of Health. *The health of elderly people: an epidemiological overview*. Central health monitoring unit epidemiological overview series, volume 1. London: HMSO.

DH 1992b Department of Health. *The health of the nation. A strategy for health in England*. London: HMSO.

DHHS 1992 Department of Health and Human Services. *Healthy people 2000*. Boston: Jones and Bartlett Publishers Inc.

DHSS 1972 Department of Health and Social Security. *A nutrition survey of the elderly*. Report on health and social subjects no. 3. London: HMSO.

DHSS 1979 Department of Health and Social Security. *Nutrition and health in old age*. Report on health and social subjects no. 16. London: HMSO.

Dickerson, J.W.T. 1988 The interrelationships of nutrition and drugs. In: *Nutrition in the clinical management of disease*. ed. Dickerson, J.W.T. and Lee, H.A. London: Edward Arnold. pp. 392–421.

Duff, K. and Hardy, J. 1995 Alzheimer's disease, mouse model made. *Nature* 373, 476–477.

Dunn, F.J. 1994 Misuse of alcohol or drugs by elderly people. *British Medical Journal* 308, 608–9.

Dunnigan, M.G. 1993 The problem with cholesterol. *British Medical Journal* 306, 1355–1356.

Durnin, J.V.G.A. and Womersley, J. 1974 Body fat assessed from total body density and its estimation from skinfold thickness: measurements on 481 men and women aged 16 to 72 years. *British Journal of Nutrition* 32, 77–97.

Echo 1993 A Department of Health newsletter. January 1993, p3.

Elmstabl, S. and Steen, B. 1987 Hospital nutrition in geriatric long term care medicine: II the effects of dietary supplements. *Age and Ageing* 16, 73–80.

Evans, J.G. 1991 Aging and rationing. *British Medical Journal* 303, 869–870.

Evans, W.J. and Meredith, C.N. 1989 Exercise and nutrition in the elderly. In: *Nutrition, aging, and the elderly.* ed. Munro, H.N. and Danford, D.E. New York: Plenum Press. pp. 89–126.

Exton-Smith, A.N. 1971 Nutrition in the elderly. *British Journal of Hospital Medicine* 5, 639–645.

Exton-Smith, A.N. 1988 Nutrition in the elderly. In: *Nutrition in the clinical management of disease.* ed. Dickerson, J.W.T. and Lee, H.A. London: Edward Arnold. pp. 110–144.

Feest, T.G., Mistry, C.D., Grimes, D.S. and Mallick, N.P. 1990 Incidence of advanced chronic renal failure and the need for end stage renal replacement therapy. *British Medical Journal* 301, 897–900.

Fenton, J. 1989 Some food for thought. *Health Service Journal* 6, 666–667.

Fiatarone, M.A. and Evans, W.J. 1993 The etiology and reversibility of muscle dysfunction in the aged. *The Journal of Gerontology* 48 (special issue), 77–83.

Fiatarone, M.A., O'Neill, E.F., Ryan, N.D., Clements, K.M., Solares, G.R., Nelson, M.E., Roberts, S.B., Kehayias, J.J., Lipsitz, L.A., Evans, W.J. 1994 Exercise training and nutritional supplementation for physical frailty in very elderly people. *The New England Journal of Medicine* 330, 1769–1775.

Fieldhouse, P. 1986 *Food and nutrition: customs and culture.* London: Croom Helm.

Freer, C. 1990 Screening the elderly *British Medical Journal* 300, 1447–1448.

Fujita, Y. 1992 Nutritional requirements of the elderly: a Japanese view. *Nutrition Reviews* 50, 449–453.

Gordon, D.J. and Rifkind, B.M. 1989 Treating high blood cholesterol in the older patient. *The American Journal of Cardiology* 63, 48h–52h.

Grant, A. and Todd, E. 1987 *Enteral and parenteral nutrition. 2nd edn.* Oxford: Blackwell Scientific Publications.

Green, R. 1994 Old age. In: *Human physiology: age, stress and the environment 2nd edn.* ed. Case, R.M. and Waterhouse, J.M. Oxford: Oxford University Press. pp. 99–123

Gregory, J., Foster, K., Tyler, H. and Wiseman, M. 1990 *The dietary and nutritional survey of British adults.* London: HMSO.

Gronbaek, M., Deis, A., Sorensen, T.I.A., Becker, U., Borch-Johnsen, K., Muller, C., Schnohr, P. and Jensen, G. 1994 Influence of sex, age, body mass index, and smoking on alcohol intake and mortality. *British Medical Journal* 308, 302–306.

Groom, H. 1993 What price a healthy diet? *The British Nutrition Foundation Nutrition Bulletin* 18, 104–109.

Grundy, E. 1992 Socio-demographic change. In: *The health of elderly people: an epidemiological overview.* Central health monitoring unit epidemiological overview series, companion papers to volume 1. London: HMSO. pp. 1–9.

Guigoz, Y., Vellas, B. and Garry, P.J. 1994 The Mini Nutritional Assessment: a practical tool for grading the nutritional state of elderly patients. *Facts and Research in Gerontology* Supplement No. 2: The mini Nutritional Assessment.

Hadfield, C. 1992 Nutritional Adequacy of a Low Protein Diet. *Journal of Renal Nutrition* 2(3) Suppl 1, 37–41.

Halliday, A. and Ashwell, M. 1991 *Non-starch polysaccharides. Briefing paper 22.* London: British Nutrition Foundation.

HEA 1994 Health Education Authority. *The balance of good health. The national food guide.* London: Health Education Authority.

Henson, S. 1992 From high street to hypermarket. Food retailing in the 1990s. In: *Your food: whose choice?* Edited by the National Consumer Council. London: HMSO. pp. 95–115.

Hill, G.L., Blackett, R.L., Pickford, I., Burkinshaw, L., Young, G.A., Warren, J.V., Schorah, C.J. and Morgan, D.B. 1977 Malnutrition in surgical patients. An unrecognised problem. *Lancet* i, 689–692.

Hubley, J. 1993 *Communicating Health – An action guide to health education and health promotion.* London: Macmillan.

Hughes, J. *et al.,*1995 The British National Diet and Nutrition Survey of people aged 65 years or over: feasibility study. *Proceedings of the Nutrition Society* published in the press – *54, 631–643.*

Hulley, S.B., Walsh, J.M.B. and Newman, T.B. 1992 Health policy on blood cholesterol time to change directions. *Circulation* 86, 1026–1029.

Isles, C.G., Hole, D.J., Gillis, C.R., Hawthorne, V.M. and Lever, A.F. 1989 Plasma cholesterol, coronary heart disease, and cancer in the Renfrew and Paisley survey. *British Medical Journal* 298, 920–924.

Jacobs, D., Blackburn, H., Higgins, M., Reed, D., Iso, H., Mcmillan, G., Neaton, J., Nelson, J., Potter, J., Rifkind, B., Rossouw, J., Shekelle, R. and Yusuf, S. 1992 Report of the conference on low blood cholesterol: mortality associations. *Circulation* 86, 1046–1059.

James, W.P.T., Ralph, A. and Sanchez-Castillo, C.P. 1987 The dominance of salt in manufactured food in the sodium intake of affluent societies. *Lancet* i, 426–428.

Jelliffe, D.B. 1967 Parallel food classifications in developing and industrialised countries. *The American Journal of Clinical Nutrition* 20, 279–281.

Jones, E., Hughes, R. and Davies, H. 1988 Intake of vitamin C and other nutrients by elderly patients receiving a hospital diet. *Journal of Human Nutrition and Dietetics* 1, 347–353.

Kanis, J.A. 1993 The incidence of hip fracture in Europe. *Osteoporosis International* 3(suppl. 1), s10–s15.

Kassianos, G. 1993 Constipation. *Care of the Elderly* 5, 444–445.

Katz, S., Branch, L.G., Branson, M.H., Papasidero, J.A., Beck, J.C. and Greer, D.S. 1983 Active life expectancy. *New England Journal of Medicine* 309, 1218–1224.

Kay, M.M.B. 1985 Immunobiology of aging. In: *Nutrition, immunity and illness in the elderly.* Chandra, R.K. ed. New York: Pergamon Press. pp. 97–119.

Keen, H. and Thomas, B. 1988 Diabetes mellitus. In: *Nutrition in the clinical management of disease.* ed. Dickerson, J.W.T. and Lee, H.A. London: Edward Arnold. pp. 167–190.

Kenney, R.A. 1989 *Physiology of aging: a synopsis.* 2nd edition. Chicago: Year Book Medical Publishers.

Keys, A., Anderson, J.T. and Grande, F. 1959 Serum cholesterol in man: diet fat and intrinsic responsiveness. *Circulation* 19, 201–204.

KFC 1992 King's Fund Centre *A positive approach to nutrition as treatment.* London: King's Fund Centre.

Kirk, S. 1990 Adequacy of meals served and consumed at a long stay hospital. *Care of the Elderly* 2, 77–80.

Klahr, S., Levey, A.S., Beck, G.J., Caggiula, A.W., Hunsicker, L., Kusek, J.W. And Striker, G. 1994 The effects of dietary protein restriction on the progression of chronic renal disease. *New England Journal Of Medicine* 330, 877–884.

Klatsky, A.L., Armstrong, M.A. and Friedman, G.D. 1992 Alcohol and mortality. *Annals of Internal Medicine* 117, 646–654.

Klipstein-Grosbuch, K., Reilly, J.J., Potter, J., Edwards, C.A. and Roberts, M.A. 1995 Energy intake and expenditure in elderly patients admitted to hospital with acute illness. *British Journal of Nutrition* 73, 323–334.

Larsson, J., Unosson, N., Ek, A.C., Ni'sson, L., Thorslund, S. and Bjurulf, P. 1990 Effect of dietary supplement on nutritional status and clinical outcome in 501 geriatric patients – a randomised study. *Clinical Nutrition* 9, 179–184.

Law, M.R., Frost, C.D. and Wald, N.J. 1991a By how much does dietary salt reduction lower blood pressure? I – Analysis of observational data among populations. *British Medical Journal* 302, 811–815.

Law, M.R., Frost, C.D. and Wald, N.J. 1991b By how much does dietary salt reduction lower blood pressure? III – Analysis of data from trials of salt reduction. *British Medical Journal* 302, 819–824.

Leather, S. 1992 Less money, less choice. Poverty and diet in the UK today. In *Your food: whose choice?* Edited by the National Consumer Council. London: HMSO. pp. 72–94.

Lee, H.A. 1988 The nutritional management of renal disease. In: *Nutrition in the clinical management of disease.* ed. Dickerson, J.W.T. and Lee, H.A. London: Edward Arnold. pp. 262–279.

Lehmann, A.B. 1991 Nutrition in old age: an update and questions for future research: part 1. *Reviews in Clinical Gerontology* 1, 135–145.

Lennard, T.W.J. and Browell, D.A. 1993 The immunological effects of trauma. *Proceedings of the Nutrition Society* 52, 85–90.

Leon, D.A. 1993 Failed or misleading adjustment for confounding. *Lancet* 342, 479–481.

Lewis, B.K., Hitchings, H., Bale, S. and Harding, K.G. 1993 Nutritional status of elderly patients with venous ulceration of the leg – report of a pilot study. *Journal of Human Nutrition and Dietetics* 6, 509–515.

McColl, K. 1988 The sugar-fat "seesaw". *The British Nutrition Foundation Nutrition Bulletin* 13, 114–118.

McCormick, J. and Skrabanek, P. 1988 Coronary heart disease is not preventable by population interventions. *Lancet* i, 839–841.

McEvoy, A.W. and James, O.F.W. 1982 The effect of a dietary supplement (Build Up) on the nutritional status of hospitalised elderly patients. *Human Nutrition: Applied Nutrition* 36A, 374–376.

McKeigue, P.M., Marmot, M.G., Adelstein, A.M., Hunt, S.P., Shipley, M.J., Butler, S.M., Riemersma, R.A. and Turner, P.R. 1985 Diet and risk factors for coronary heart disease in Asians in northwest London. *Lancet* ii, 1086–1089.

McKeigue, P.M., Shah, B. and Marmot, M.G. 1991 Relation of central obesity and insulin resistance with high diabetes prevalence and cardiovascular risk in South Asians. *Lancet* 337, 382–386.

Macnair, A.L. 1994 Physical activity, not diet, should be the focus of measures for the primary prevention of cardiovascular disease. *Nutrition Research Reviews* 7, 43–65.

McWhirter, J.P. and Pennington, C.R. 1994 Incidence and recognition of malnutrition in hospital. *British Medical Journal* 308, 945–948.

MAFF Ministry of Agriculture Fisheries and Food 1993 *National food survey 1992* London: HMSO.

Marsh, A.G., Sanchez, T.V., Michelsen, O., Chaffee, F.L. and Fagal, S.M. 1988 Vegetarian lifestyle and bone mineral density. *American Journal of Clinical Nutrition* 48, 837–841.

Martin, J., Meltzer, H. and Elliot, D. 1988 *OPCS surveys of disability in Great Britain Report 1*. London: HMSO.

Maslow, A.H. 1943 A theory of human motivation. *Psychological Reviews* 50, 370–396.

Mattila, K., Haavisto, M. and Rajala, S. 1986 Body mass index and mortality in the elderly. *British Medical Journal* 292, 867–868.

Mattson, F.H. and Grundy, S.M. 1985 Comparison of effects of dietary saturated, monounsaturated and polyunsaturated fatty acids on plasma lipids and lipoproteins in man. *Journal of Lipid Research* 26, 194–202.

Mensink, R.P. and Katan, M.J. 1990 Effect of dietary trans fatty acids on high-density and low-density lipoprotein cholesterol levels in healthy subjects. *The New England Journal of Medicine* 323, 439–445.

Morgan, D.B. and Schorah, C.J. 1986 Nutrition and the mental state of the elderly. In: *Psychiatric disorders in the elderly*. Bebbington, P.E. and Jacoby, R. eds. London: Mental Health Foundation. pp. 75–89.

Morris, J.N., Everitt, M.G., Pollard, R., Chave, S.P.W. and Semmence, A.M. 1980 Vigorous exercise in leisure-time: protection against coronary heart disease. *Lancet* ii, 1207–1210.

Mowe, M., Bohmer, T. and Kindt, E. 1994 Reduced nutritional status in elderly people is probable before disease and probably contributes to the development of disease. *American Journal of Clinical Nutrition* 59, 317–324.

NACNE 1983 The National Advisory Committee on Nutrition Education. *A discussion paper on proposals for nutritional guidelines for health education in Britain*. London: Health Education Council.

NAGE British Dietetic Association/Nutrition Advisory Group for Elderly People 1992 *Eating through the 90s*. Leeds: NAGE

NAGE British Dietetic Association /Nutrition Advisory Group for Elderly People 1994 *Dietetic standards of care for the older adult in hospital. Leeds: NAGE*.

Nahas, A.M.E. and Coles, G.A. 1986 Dietary treatment of chronic renal failure: ten unanswered questions. *Lancet* i, 597–600.

Neaton, J.D., Blackburn, H., Jacobs, D., Kuller, L., Lee, D-J., Sherwin, R., Shih, J., Stamler, J. and Wentworth, D. 1992 Serum cholesterol level and mortality findings for men screened in the mutiple risk factor intervention trial. *Archives of Internal Medicine* 152, 1490–1500.

Newton, H. Schorah, C.J., Habibzadeh, N., Morgan, D.B. and Hullin, R.P. 1985 The cause and correction of low blood vitamin C concentrations in the elderly. *American Journal of Clinical Nutrition* 42, 656–659.

NOS National Osteoporosis Society 1993 *Osteoporosis – a guide to its causes, treatment and prevention.* Radstock, Bath: National Osteoporosis Society.

NRC 1989a National Research Council. *Recommended dietary allowances.* 10th edn. Washington D.C.: National Academy of Sciences.

NRC 1989b National Research Council. Diet and health: implications for reducing chronic disease risk. *Nutrition Reviews* 47, 142–149.

Oliver, M.F. 1981 Diet and coronary heart disease. *British Medical Bulletin* 37, 49–58.

OPCS Office of Population Censuses and Surveys 1991 *Mortality statistics: cause 1990.* London: HMSO.

OPCS Office of Population Censuses and Surveys 1993 *Mortality statistics: deaths by cause, age and sex 1992* London: HMSO.

Paffenbarger, R.S., Hyde, R.T., Wing, A.L. and Hsieh, C-C. 1986 Physical activity, all cause mortality, and longevity of college alumni. *New England Journal of Medicine* 314, 605–613.

Penn, N.D., Purkins, L., Kelleher, R.V., Heatley, R.V., Mascie-Taylor, B.H. and Belfield, P.W. 1991 The effect of dietary supplementation with vitamins A, C and E on cell-mediated immune function in elderly long-stay patients: a randomised control trial. *Age and Ageing* 20, 169–174.

Prentice, A.M., Leavesley, K., Murgatroyd,P.R., Coward,W.A., Schorah, C.T., Bladon, R.P. and Hullin, R.P. 1989 Is severe wasting in elderly mental patients caused by an excessive energy requirement? *Age and Ageing* 18, 158–167.

Prior, J. 1992 A project to assess and improve nutritional provision at a care of the elderly unit. *Care of the Elderly* 4, 244–248.

RCN Royal College of Nursing 1993 *Nutrition standards and the older adult.* Dynamic Quality Improvement Programme. London: RCN.

Reilly, J.J., Mackintosh, M., Potter, J. and Roberts, M.A. 1995 An evaluation of the feasibility of sip-feed supplementation in undernourished, acutely sick, elderly patients. *Proceedings of the Nutrition Society* 54, 135A.

Roberts, D. 1982 Factors contributing to outbreaks of food poisoning in England and Wales 1970–1979. *Journal of Hygiene.* Cambridge 89, 491–498.

Robertson, I., Glekin, B.M., Henderson, J.B., Lakhani, A. and Dunnigan, M.G. 1982 Nutritional deficiencies amongst ethnic minorities in the United Kingdom. *Proceedings of the Nutrition Society* 41, 243–256.

Robins, A. and Wittenberg, R. 1992 In: *The health of elderly people: an epidemiological overview.* Central health monitoring unit epidemiological overview series, companion papers to volume 1. London: HMSO. pp. 10–19.

Roe, D.A. 1993 Drug-nutrient interactions. In Garrow, J.S. and James, W.P.T. eds. *Human nutrition and dietetics. 9th edn.* Edinburgh: Churchill Livingstone. pp.761–766.

Rolls, B.J. and Phillips, P.A. 1990 Aging and disturbances of thirst and fluid balance. *Nutrition Reviews* 48, 137–144.

Rudman, D. 1988 Kidney Senescence; A model for aging. *Nutrition Reviews* 46, 209.

Sanders, T.A.B. 1985 Influence of fish-oil supplements on man. *Proceedings of the Nutrition Society* 44, 391–397.

Schroll, M., Jorgensen, L., Osler, M. and Davidsen, M. 1993 Chronic undernutrition and the aged. *Proceedings of the Nutrition Society* 52, 29–37.

Seidell, J.C. 1992 Regional obesity and health. *International Journal of Obesity* 16(suppl 2), S31–S34.

Simpson, H.C.R. 1981 High-carbohydrate, high-fibre diets for diabetics. *Proceedings of the Nutrition Society* 40, 219–225.

Shipley, M.J., Pocock, S.J. and Marmot, M.G. 1991 Does plasma cholesterol concentration predict mortality from coronary heart disease in elderly people? 18 year follow up in the Whitehall study. *British Medical Journal* 303, 89–92.

Simon, S. 1991 A survey of the nutritional adequacy of meals served and eaten by patients. *Nursing Practice pages* 7–11.

Sizer, F. and Whitney, H. 1994 *Hamilton and Whitney's Nutrition concepts and controversies 6th edn.* St Paul, Mn: West Publishing Co.

Sjogren, A., Osterberg, T. and Steen, B. 1994 Intake of energy, nutrients and food items in a ten–year cohort comparison and in a six–year longitudinal perspective: A population study of 70 and 76 year old Swedish people. *Age and Ageing* 23, 108–112.

Smith, G.D., Song, F. and Sheldon, T.A. 1993 Cholesterol lowering and mortality: the importance of considering initial level of risk. *British Medical Journal* 306, 1367–1373.

Smith, R. 1987 Osteoporosis: cause and management. *British Medical Journal* 294, 329–332.

Spector, T.D., Cooper, C. and Fenton Lewis, A. 1990 Trends in admissions for hip fracture in England and Wales 1968–1985. *British Medical Journal* 300, 1173–1174.

Steen, B. The changing face of ageing. In: *The health of elderly people: an epidemiological overview.* Central health monitoring unit epidemiological overview series, companion papers to volume 1. London: HMSO. pp. 36–43.

Taylor, S. and Goodinson–McClaren, S. 1992 *Nutritional support: a team approach.* London: Wolfe Publishing.

Thomas, B. 1994 *The Manual of Dietetic Practice 2nd edn* London: Blackwell Scientific Publications.

Thompson, K. 1993 Screening strategy takes hold. *Care of the Elderly* 5, 290.

Thurnham, D. 1992 Micronutrients: how important in old age? *European Journal of Clinical Nutrition* 46(suppl. 3), S29–S37.

Todd, E.A., Hunt, P., Crowe, P.T. and Royle, G.T. 1984 What do patients eat in hospital? *Human Nutrition: Applied Nutrition* 38A, 294–297.

Tomkins, A. and Watson, F. 1989 *Malnutrition and infection. A review.* London: Clinical Nutrition Unit, London School of Hygiene and Tropical Medicine.

USDA 1992 United States Department of Agriculture. *The food guide pyramid*. Home and garden bulletin number 252. Washington DC: United States Department of Agriculture.

Webb, G.P. 1992 A critical survey of methods used to investigate links between diet and disease. *Journal of Biological Education,* 26(4), 263–271.

Webb, G.P. 1994 A survey of fifty years of dietary standards 1943–1993. *Journal of Biological Education* 28(i), 101–108.

Webb, G.P. 1995 *Nutrition: a health promotion approach.* London: Edward Arnold.

White, A., Nicolaas, G., Foster, K., Browne, F. and Carey, S. 1993 *Health survey for England* 1991 London: HMSO.

Wickham, C.A.C., Walsh, K., Barker, D.J.P., Margetts, B.M., Morris, J. and Bruce, S.A. 1989 Dietary calcium, Physical activity, and risk of hip fracture: a prospective study. *British Medical Bulletin* 299, 889–892.

Willet, W.C., Stampfer, M.J., Manson, J.E., Colditz, G.A., Speizer, F.E., Rosner, B.A., Sampson, L.A. and Hennekens, C.H. 1993 Intake of trans fatty acids and risk of coronary heart disease among women. *Lancet* 341, 581–585.

Woo, J., Ho, S.C., Mak, Y.T., Law, L.K. and Cheung, A. 1994 Nutritional status of elderly people during recovery from chest infection and the role of nutritional supplementation assessed by a prospective randomized single-blind control trial. *Age and Ageing* 23, 40–48.

Recommended reading

Chandra, R.K. (ed) 1985 *Nutrition, immunity and illness in the elderly*. New York: Pergamon Press. A multi-author compilation of specialist reviews.

COMA 1992 Committee on Medical Aspects of Food Policy. *The nutrition of elderly people*. Report on health and social subjects no. 43. London: HMSO. A review of the major issues with many practical recommendations and recommendations for further research.

The Caroline Walker Trust 1995 *Eating well for older people*. London: The Caroline Walker Trust. A practical guide for those involved in catering for the elderly.

Department of Health 1992. *The health of elderly people: an epidemiological overview*. Central health monitoring unit epidemiological overview series, volume 1. London: HMSO. A mine of statistical information on the health of elderly Britons.

Department of Health 1992 *The health of elderly people: an epidemiological overview*. Central health monitoring unit epidemiological overview series, companion papers to volume 1. London: HMSO. A series of specialist papers discussing the implications of some of the above statistical information.

Green, R. 1994 Old age. In: *Human physiology: age, stress and the environment* 2nd edn. ed. Case, R.M. and Waterhouse, J.M. Oxford: Oxford University Press. pp.99-123. A brief review of the physiological effects of ageing.

Kenney, R.A. 1989 *Physiology of aging: a synopsis*. 2nd edition. Chicago: Year Book Medical Publishers. A more substantial review of the physiological effects of ageing.

Munro, H.N. and Danford, D.E. (eds.) 1989 *Nutrition, aging, and the elderly*. New York: Plenum Press. A multi-author compilation of specialists reviews.

RCN Royal College of Nursing (1993) *Nutrition standards and the older adult*. Dynamic Quality Improvement Programme. London: RCN. Particularly useful on nutritional assessment in the elderly.

Webb, G.P. 1995 *Nutrition: a health promotion approach*. London: Edward Arnold. Recommended for those with limited background in nutrition.

Index